Success
Beyond
Work

**What Prosperous
Massage Therapists Know—
Minimum Work,
Maximum Profits, and
a Sellable Business**

Colleen (Steigerwald) Holloway, LMT

Saramore Publishing Company
GRASONVILLE, MARYLAND

First printing 2003

ISBN 0-9722939-4-9
LCCN 2002110167

ATTENTION CORPORATIONS, UNIVERSITIES, COLLEGES, AND PROFESSIONAL ORGANIZATIONS: Quantity discounts are available on bulk purchases of this book for educational, gift purposes, or as premiums for increasing magazine subscriptions or renewals. Special books or book excerpts can also be created to fit specific needs. For information, please contact Saramore Publishing Company, 802 Oyster Cove Drive, Grasonville, MD 21638; ph. 410-827-4281.

CONTENTS

ACKNOWLEDGMENTS

To the most loving, giving people I know...my parents, for standing behind me each time I stood out on a ledge. You did all of the worrying for me.

To the man of my dreams...my wonderful husband, David, who believed in me and supported me, even when I lost sight of the end of the rainbow.

INTRODUCTION

Have you ever dreamed of owning a successful massage therapy business? Or do you already have your own business but feel you've reached a financial plateau and don't know how to generate more income without working even more hours? If you've answered "yes" to either of these questions, accept that fate has landed this book into your hands, for within you will find the answers to guide you to financial success.

The creation of this book was inspired by one of your fellow colleagues—me. After graduating from massage therapy school in 1991 and passing the state licensing examination, I ventured out to begin a career in the massage therapy field. I relocated from Long Island to my hometown of Saratoga Springs, New York.

Here, I began looking for a place to work. I considered working for a spa but felt it would limit my abilities and income. I called two local chiropractors, arranged for a meeting, and soon after began working in their offices as an independent contractor. I also found work at a local printing plant, hair salon, and counseling center. I was determined to support myself in the field I loved.

For one year, I worked in these five locations, building my clientele and reputation. I then decided to take the leap and rent space for an office. I called a few other massage therapists and asked them to join me as independent contractors. Professional Massage Associates was established.

After nine years in business, with a staff of eight, I decided to relocate to another state. I felt in my heart I couldn't just leave my business or close it, so I decided to sell it. Two years later, I sold the business—for a six-figure price tag.

During the two years I was trying to sell the business, I discovered that most massage therapists have little or no equity in their business, and therefore, cannot sell their business when they decide they no longer want to do massage. Most simply just close their doors and walk away with nothing to show for their years of dedicated work.

I decided to find a means of helping my colleagues to profit from their years of dedicated, hard work. This book will be of value to you no matter where you are in your massage career, whether you are just beginning, looking to increase your clientele and earn more money, or seeking to end your career. It will take you through the necessary steps, from establishing your business to selling it, and to achieving ultimate financial success. Even if you practice massage out of your home, this book will teach you what steps to take to build enough equity to make your business profitable and sellable.

This book is separated into four parts: (1) establish your business, (2) market your business, (3) build equity, and (4) profit from your business. It is important to follow each section in order and not to skip any parts. Even if your business is well established, go through each part because there is important information in each section that is necessary in creating a successful and sellable business.

Part I

Establish
Your Business

Setting up a successful massage therapy business requires making many important decisions, including where you will practice, what you will charge, and what services you will offer. Many of your decisions will have a long-term effect on your business, so they need to be well thought out. The first two chapters cover the decisions that will have the greatest impact on your level of success.

CHAPTER ONE

Setting Up Your Practice

LOCATION, LOCATION, LOCATION!

Selecting the proper location for your business is the first important step in creating a successful operation. To start this process, contact your local economic development office to obtain information on zoning laws and ask if any business licenses or permits are required. Once you've gathered this information, you will be ready to search for a location.

In choosing a suitable location, take into consideration the following questions:

- Is the location easy to find? Write down the directions you would give a new client and decide if they could easily find it.
- Is there adequate, easily accessible, and well-lit parking for your clients?
- Is the space handicap accessible? The American Disabilities Act, passed by Congress in 1990, requires proper accessibility. Think about the clients you will be treating. Can they easily maneuver in this location? Are there stairs to climb?
- What about walk-ins? Is that possible in this location?
- Would you feel safe working in this location? At night?
- Do other local businesses have similar hours as you?
- What safety measures are in place, such as security systems and locking mechanisms?

4

- Is the space quiet? Make sure there isn't a dentist drilling teeth or a grief counseling center with yelling patients next door. What about street noise? Is there a business located above you?
- What about ventilation? If your location is in a professional building, you could be smelling another tenant's lunch every day if the ventilation system is poor.
- Is there adequate water available (at least one sink and a toilet)? If you're thinking of doing water treatments or laundry, determine the amount of hot water you will be using.
- Are there adequate electrical outlets in each room for your needs?
- What about the temperature controls? Can you adjust them or will you need to find other means of keeping your clients comfortable?
- Is there a building manager for repairs or emergencies? If not, who will be taking care of maintenance problems?
- Is there room to grow your business in this location or will you need to relocate in the future?

If the location is in a professional building, talk to the other tenants to see how they like their location and landlord. Ask them if maintenance problems are handled within a reasonable time.

Think of yourself as a client entering this location. Would you feel comfortable here, or would you rather go someplace else? If you would rather go someplace else, keep looking for another location.

You may consider talking with a real estate agent who deals with commercial leasing or commercial properties for sale (if you're looking to buy your location). They can help facilitate the process of finding the perfect location for your new business.

NAMING YOUR BUSINESS

Once you find the perfect location for your business, you need to create a name for it. You may decide to use your own name as the business name or create a different name. Whatever you choose, consider the following:

- You will be reciting the name on the telephone, so make sure it is easy to pronounce and not too lengthy.
- Since Yellow Pages advertising is alphabetical, where will your advertising fall? This is especially important if you live in a large city with a lot of massage therapists. You'll want to choose a name that begins with A, B, or C to place your advertisement at the top of the listings.
- What do you want to convey about your business within the name? Is it "professional," "relaxing," "therapeutic," and so forth?
- Will you have other professionals working in your location? If so, you may want to use "associates," "alliance," or "association" in your business name.
- If you are planning on offering several different services in your business, be cautious about using the word "massage" in your business name, for it will sound like all you offer is massage when you may also offer acupuncture, hydrotherapy, and skin care.

Whatever name you choose for your business name, be sure to register it locally at the county clerk's office, if you are required to do so. This will protect your business name from being used by someone else.

BUSINESS STRUCTURE

Your new business will need to be structured for both liability and tax purposes. Therefore, you will need to register it as one of the following:

- *Sole proprietor*: One person operates the business as an individual. This is the most common type of business structure for a massage therapy business. All business profits are taxed as income to the owner. The owner has control of all business decisions but holds complete responsibility for liability of its debts. To become a sole proprietor, one applies for a business permit at the county clerk's office in the county in which the business is located.

- *Partnership*: Two or more people join together to operate the business. Here, a formal partnership agreement is necessary. Regardless of your relationship with your partner(s), do not become a partnership without an agreement that addresses the duties, decision processes, and expectations of each partner. A lawyer is recommended for forming the agreement. Each partner shares liability for all debts of the business. All profits are taxed as income to the partners, based on their percentages of ownership. To become a partnership, one applies for a business permit at the county clerk's office in the county in which the business is located.

- *C corporation*: This is the most complex form of business structure in which there are shareholders, directors, and officers. There are more government regulations here and profits are subject to double taxation. There is limited liability but not total protection from liability. In most cases, a massage therapy business would not benefit from this structure.

- *S corporation*: This structure regulates like the C corporation but it permits a corporation's profits to be taxed as a sole proprietorship or partnership. To qualify for this structure, a business must meet certain requirements. For more information, contact the IRS to request IRS publication 589.

- *Limited liability company (LLC)*: This is becoming a popular business structure. This type of business combines both corporate and partnership characteristics. There is more flexibility in operating the business than a corporation and owners have limited liability. Personal assets are not at risk.

Unless you are an expert in this field, I recommend you consult an accountant for assistance in choosing the business structure best suited for your business.

FACILITY AND LAYOUT

Facility

A massage therapy business should minimally consist of one treatment room, a bathroom, a reception area, and storage space. A small office is also ideal but not necessary to establish your business. As your business grows, you will need a larger space with additional treatments rooms. But for now, you'll need just the minimal space for your business—at least 400 square feet to start. Let's look at each room individually, before designing your layout.

Treatment room: The optimal size for a treatment room is 10 feet by 12 feet. If your space is too small or too large, your client will not feel comfortable. If it is too small, you will not be able to move freely. If you can open the door and touch the table without stepping into the room, it is too small. A window is desirable, especially if the room is small. A faucet and sink are also recommended in the room for sanitary purposes. Your clients will be relieved to know your hands are clean if they see you wash your hands before and after the treatment.

Bathroom: A bathroom is necessary for obvious reasons. Make sure it is well stocked with the essentials (toilet paper, paper towels, soap, and so forth). If your business is located in a professional building, you may have a communal bathroom just outside your office space. This is great because you don't have to pay for the space; however, make sure it is convenient for you and your client to get to and that it is clean. But if you are thinking of offering water treatments, you will need a bathroom within your space. You do not want your clients walking down the hall of the building in a robe!

Reception area: Your reception area should, of course, be a comfortable space for your clients to relax and fill out information forms. It should be large enough to accommodate your client load, with at least six seating spaces. There also needs to be space for retail (which you will learn more about in later chapters of this book). This can consist of shelves on the wall, if your space is small. You will also need a reception area to check out your clients and answer the telephone. This can be a desk or a counter.

Storage space: You'll need a space to store linens (both clean and soiled), stereo and equipment, office supplies, cleaning supplies, extra retail, blankets, refrigerator, microwave, copier, and so forth. Make sure you have at least one closet. Some massage tables come with cabinets beneath them for added storage, but you will still need a closet.

Layout

The level of noise and distractions within your facility will depend largely on the positioning of each room and is an important consideration when creating a peaceful environment. Usually the *reception room* is the first room you see upon entering a massage therapy business. If possible, the *bathroom* is best located just off the reception room, so your clients can use it prior to their appointment without disturbing other clients who are receiving treatments. If the bathroom is located next to the treatment room, your clients may be distracted by the sound of the toilet flushing and running water. The *storage space*, however, can be located almost anywhere, but is best situated in an area away from any treatment rooms.

The *treatment room* needs to be located in the quietest place, furthest from the reception room, telephone, and outer environmental noise. In the field of massage therapy, a quiet environment is essential for both relaxation and healing.

ENVIRONMENT

Environment can be defined as "the totality of surrounding conditions." Because there are many influences involved in creating your business environment, it is very important. Many therapists don't spend enough time planning this portion of their massage business. Just think for a moment. Have you ever received a massage in a place where you just couldn't relax? Or have you ever walked into a massage business and felt uncomfortable immediately? Think from your clients' perspective. They will be undressing and then allowing you to touch them, often for the first time. You want your clients to feel at ease, safe, and relaxed from the moment they enter your business until they exit.

To create a magnificent environment, you will need to use all of the five senses of the body: visual, auditory, kinesthetic, olfactory, and gustatory. Let's look at each of the senses individually.

Visual (seeing): What does the client see in your office that is visually pleasing? Is the lighting soft to create the feel of warmth? Are there educational posters and brochures that emphasize professionalism and knowledge? How about fresh flowers and plants? These offer comfort and emulate life. Are the walls painted a warm color or are they stark white? Do the walls have pictures of beautiful scenery that give a sense of serenity?

Auditory (hearing): What are some of the sounds your clients hear that bring a sense of relaxation? Is there soft music playing that will immediately slow their minds down. Do you have a water fountain or fish tank in the reception area and/or treatment room to subdue their thoughts? How about a sound machine of happy birds singing or a babbling brook? Soft wind chimes just inside the reception door ring peace and tranquility.

Kinesthetic (feeling): What do your clients "feel" that brings them comfort? You may have a great touch, but are your hands warm when you touch your client or do you torture them with cold hands and then apologize? My hands were always cold in the wintertime, so I made sure to wash them in hot water before the treatment, then warmed my massage oil in the microwave or in a bottle warmer and wrapped my hands around the bottle before touching the client. Clients often asked, "How did you get your hands so warm? That feels good."

Are there soft floors or rugs to walk on? How about warmth? If your clients are not warm throughout their massage, the entire experience will be a bad one. Do you have flannel sheets in the winter? Or do you use an electric mattress pad on the table? Although some therapists don't like the "energy" of an electric blanket, my clients loved it throughout the year. Is there air conditioning in the summer? It is amazing how the little things you do for your clients make such a big difference.

Olfactory (smelling): Smells can be pleasant and calming or bothersome and unpleasant, so be careful when creating this sense. Upon entering your business, fresh flowers can bring smiles to faces. I always had a few fresh flowers in a vase on my desk and almost every client who sat there had their nose in them. How about a vanilla candle in the treatment or reception area? You could place a lavender pillow on your client's eyes.

You can use aromatherapy in any room by applying scented oil to a "scented ball" outlet or you can add aroma oil to your massage oil or lotion. If you're going to do this, I recommend you have a bottle of unscented oil and a few bottles of scented combined oils— maybe an uplifting oil and a relaxing oil—your clients can choose from. If you wanted to do something really special and personalized, you could blend a specific oil for each client.

Gustatory (tasting): What do you offer your clients to eat or drink that is pleasurable? Do you have a water cooler? You know we all recommend our clients drink a lot of water after their massage. Maybe you could pour your client a glass of water and add a lemon wedge, and place it in the treatment room just after the massage. How about offering herbal teas or juice to enjoy after the treatment? Are there breath mints in the treatment room? What about a bowl of wrapped candy placed in the reception room during the holidays, or a bowl of fresh apples? You don't have to be extravagant here but find some means of adding this sense to your environment.

Each of the five senses needs to be used in all rooms within your business. Don't limit your creative, warm environment to just the treatment room. The environment should flow from room to room, throughout your business.

THE RECEPTIONIST

You may be thinking you don't need (or can't afford) to hire a receptionist. Let me tell you from experience that you won't be able to get where you are aimed at going by doing everything yourself. Although you may save some money, it won't be long before you find yourself worn down, working long hours with little time to do the things your business truly needs in order for you to be successful. Hence, you will need to hire what I call a "multi-task" person to assist you. This person may start out assisting you for five to ten hours a week, then move into full-time employment, depending on what phase your business is in and how fast it grows. You may also think about bartering massage treatments in exchange for these services.

The multi-tasker will be busy every moment you employ him or her. The primary function of this position is to be your receptionist. The person who warmly greets your clients and has them fill out information forms. The person who also answers the telephone, schedules appointments, answers questions, and sells retail and gift certificates. This person will take care of all aspects of your laundry, whether it calls for sorting, folding, ordering, or washing. He or she will pull your daily client charts and file them, inventory your retail and order more when needed, prepare marketing mailings, water your plants, clean the office, prepare your treatment room for the next client, and so forth. Before you hire a receptionist, consult your state employment office for information on the legal requirements of having an employee, such as tax withholdings.

If your business is going to be successful, you must learn to delegate the things that do not generate income to you and get focused on building equity in your business.

MISSION STATEMENT

What is a mission statement? And why do you need one? A mission statement defines the intent for your business. It states what your goals are and is beneficial not only to you, but also to your clients. How can you possibly promote your business if you can't clearly communicate what it is?

A mission statement should be a one-sentence, clear, concise statement that says what the business is and what it aims to do. In other words, it is a simple public relations statement, easy to remember and repeat, that you and your staff can effectively use to promote your business. For example, my mission statement for writing this book is, "A guide for teaching massage therapists how to create a successful business that is both profitable and sellable." My goal is to educate and prepare those who are entering the massage therapy business and those who are currently operating massage therapy businesses on how to structure their business so they can build equity and in turn have income from the sale of their business when they choose to retire from it.

In preparing the mission statement for your business, think of what words will portray your intent, such as "relax, soothe, heal, nurture, indulge, balance." Here's an example of another mission statement: "Healing Hands…staffed with the highest credentials, we offer innovative healing treatments to calm your spirit and soothe your soul."

Your mission statement can be displayed in your reception area for your clients to read, as well as in your advertising materials, such as your brochure. Think of it as a constant reminder of what your business stands for and what its main objective is.

CHAPTER TWO

Operations

POLICIES

Establishing good policies for your business will help you to operate it successfully. Policies set guidelines for the business owner to provide good customer service. They also inform the consumer of any rules you have in place.

The following are some policies for you to consider establishing.

Appointment Cancellation Policy

A written policy needs to be in place for appointment cancellations. If you do not have this policy, you will endure last-minute cancellations from clients, which will in turn cost you money. You will also be losing clients you turned away for an appointment when you could have seen them. Your time is valuable because you can see only so many clients per day. Having one last-minute cancellation per week can reduce your annual income by thousands of dollars!

I recommend an appointment cancellation policy of twenty-four-hour notice to cancel the appointment, unless there is a valid emergency, such as an illness or vehicle breakdown.

There are several ways to convey your policy to your clients. I recommend using all of them.

- State your policy in writing. Place a typed notice in a picture frame in your reception area that reads, "Our time together is important. Unless there is an emergency, we request that you cancel your appointment 24 hours in advance or pay the missed appointment fee in full."

- On your business appointment cards, have printed under the time and date, a line that reads "24 hours' notice required for cancellation."
- The above line should also be printed on all brochures and rate cards.
- When first-time clients make an appointment, verbally inform them of your cancellation policy.

As a general rule, I do not charge a client for the first appointment that is missed or canceled without notice. I do, however, inform them again of my policy and tell them that I will need to charge them if a future appointment is missed or canceled without proper notice. I then place a note in their chart that they missed one appointment. This is a courtesy rule that works well for me. It waives the charge for the client one time, while giving them a warning that the policy will be upheld in the future.

When a client misses a second appointment, I call and explain that I am sorry he or she missed the appointment but I will need to charge for it. Your clients will respect you if you show them you are a professional businessperson. If they don't, refer them elsewhere for you do not need a client who does not value your time.

Some massage therapists call their clients a day or two in advance to remind them of their upcoming appointment. This suggestion will help to decrease missed appointments. Or, when making appointments for clients, ask if they would like a reminder call. Some will and some won't.

Lateness Policy

A written policy needs to be established to deal with clients who are late for their appointments. Without this policy, you will place yourself in an awkward position of giving the late client their full scheduled time, leaving you late with your next "on-time" client or cutting the appointment time short and having your late client become upset.

To state your policy in writing, place a typed notice in a picture frame in your reception area and/or treatment room that reads, "We request that you arrive early for your appointment. In order for us to uphold our professional standards of being 'on time,' we regret that we cannot give you additional time if you arrive late for your appointment. If for any reason *we* are late starting your appointment, you will receive the full scheduled time."

Note that to adhere to this policy, it is essential for you to allow a minimum of 15 minutes between each appointment for you to reset the treatment room.

Both the cancellation and lateness policy can also be printed together as a form, or at the bottom of the health intake form your new client will fill out, and then signed by your client.

BUSINESS HOURS

Having set business hours will give the business a more professional image and will also omit your having to be available 24/7. Some therapists who don't establish set hours have to deal with clients calling at all hours wanting an appointment. Also, if you do not establish business hours you will find yourself working long hours with gaps in your schedule.

While setting business hours, consider working a varied schedule to accommodate client schedules. As an example you could work two mornings and two evenings and alternate Saturday or Sundays. Once you set your business hours, you will need to adhere to them because steady clients will want their "regular" appointment time each week.

If your business is already established and you have other therapists working for you, it is a good idea to alternate therapists' schedules so more business hours are available.

Once you have established your business hours, print them on your brochures and rate cards. Also record them on your answering machine or voicemail.

FEES

How much should you charge for your services? First, you need to determine the length of time of each treatment that you will offer—30 minutes, 45 minutes, 60 minutes, 75 minutes, 90 minutes, and so forth. Next, call numerous massage businesses in your area to find out what their fees are. With this information, you can better decide what is fair to charge for your services. If you establish fees higher than your competitors', your services must warrant the higher fees. On the other hand, if your fees are lower than your competitors', you may not be respected as a qualified professional.

Once your fees are established, put them in writing, either in a brochure or on a rate card. Post them in your reception area—perhaps typed and placed in an attractive picture frame. Some states require that fees for services are posted.

I raised my fees every two years, by about $5. When you choose to raise your fees will be determined by your competitors' fee increases and how well your business is doing. When it does come time to raise your fees, it's a good idea to let your clients know about 30 days in advance. You can place a typed announcement in a picture frame in the reception area and also tell them as they make future appointments with you. I had only a few clients who "complained" about price increases. Because they were such loyal clients, I kept them at the old rate and they appreciated it. The decision is always yours to make on an individual basis.

METHODS OF PAYMENT

How will your clients pay for your services and products? Although cash is always an acceptable method of payment, will you also accept checks? What about out-of-state checks? How about credit and/or debit cards?

I have always accepted local checks. In my 10 years of business, I can count only a handful of checks that "bounced." When this happened, I would call the client and have them pay all of the expenses I incurred because of the returned check. I did not have a policy for charging a client a "bounced check fee" because I believed clients felt bad enough about the check not clearing. You may, however, choose to establish a check policy with a fee for returned checks. If you decide to do so, type your policy notice (fee included) and place it in a picture frame in your reception area.

Choosing whether or not to offer credit and debit cards as a method of payment depends largely on the size of your business. If you are a small, one-person business you may not need to accept this method of payment yet. But if you are a larger business, I recommend accepting credit and debit cards.

Accepting credit and debit cards will generate more income to your business. Clients are more inclined to get a massage and purchase products and gift certificates if they don't have to pay immediately. Also, accepting credit cards will greatly increase your gift certificate sales, since clients can purchase them over the telephone. (For more information about gift certificates, see page 38.)

On the downside, you will have to pay service charges for accepting credit and debit cards. Check with your bank where your business checking account is, to find out how to become a credit card merchant and what the fees will be. There is typically a set monthly service fee, as well as a percentage fee per credit card dollar amount, which is usually between 2 and 5 percent. In addition, there is sometimes a small rental fee for the credit card equipment to scan with. You can shop around for competitive rates by looking in your local Yellow Pages under "Credit Card Plans/Services."

You will need to weigh the costs of having the service with the benefits of increased income. Again, most businesses will increase their income by offering this service.

If you do choose this method of payment, make sure your printed advertising materials reflect your payment options, especially your Yellow Pages advertising.

DESIGNING YOUR MENU

Your printed menu of services will list what services you offer, a brief description of each treatment, and the prices. This is a good time to become creative with your services perhaps by offering a "signature" treatment such as a head-to-toe treatment consisting of an aromatherapy face and scalp massage followed by foot reflexology and completed with a warm paraffin foot dip. Decide what is unique about your business and then convey it. Use words such as warm, healing, professional, therapeutic, relaxing, soothing, and so forth to describe the business and be sure to include the mission statement you created earlier in this chapter (see page 12).

Some therapists offer a discounted package on a series of treatments. If you are just beginning your business, this may be a good way to entice new clients to become regulars. But keep your discount very small or you will decrease your income too much. If you are already established with clientele, I do not recommend a discounted package. Your regular clients who would come anyway will simply be paying less money to you.

If the only service you offer is massage, list all the types of massage you offer, such as Swedish, shiatsu, tai, amma, neuromuscular therapy, myofascial release, lymphatic drainage, prenatal, infant, aromatherapy, cranio-sacral therapy, hot rock massage, foot reflexology, and so forth. This will enhance the appearance of your level of expertise more than simply stating "massage."

Other professional services to offer that complement massage include steam, sauna, hydrotherapy (baths), manicure, pedicure, facials, paraffin treatments, salt glows/body wraps, yoga classes, Pilates, chiropractic, physical therapy, and acupuncture. These services require a separate license or certification in many states, which you could obtain yourself or hire another professional to perform.

When printing your material, make sure it can fit into a regular-sized envelop for mailings and display racks. Remember to keep the information (1) simple, (2) enticing, and (3) inviting. Be sure to add your business name, address, telephone number, email, Web address, and a map or directions to your location. Also mention that gift certificates are available and which credit cards are accepted, if that applies.

I recommend printing 500 pieces of material at a time because your menu of services can change, especially if your business is growing, and your prices will eventually increase. (See the sample menu in Appendix B, page 79.)

CLIENT INTAKE FORM

It is essential to have a general form for your clients to fill out upon their first visit. From this form you will gather information on any contraindications for treatment, as well as the areas you will need to focus on. You will also obtain the client's name, address, and telephone information, which is useful for future mailings and appointment reminders.

It is also recommended that you retain information on each client as they return to your business for appointments; and in some states, it is mandatory that you retain health records. You can begin taking notes on the back of the client intake form by writing the date of each treatment followed by any comments about the treatment or condition of the client. You can continue notetaking on additional paper, as needed. For a more professional medical business, some therapists use SOAP notes for recordkeeping. SOAP (Subjective, Objective, Assessment, Plan) notes are a professional, medical method of note taking. Whatever direction your business will lean toward, whether it be medical/therapeutic or spa/relaxing, will determine the type of records you will maintain.

You may want to ask your clients, upon each returning visit to your business, if their address and telephone number have changed, and if any of their medical information has changed. This will keep your records current. (See the sample client intake form in Appendix B, page 75.)

INSURANCE COVERAGE

There are several types of insurance to consider when establishing your business; you will need them until you retire. There are three types of insurance all massage therapists *must* have to protect themselves and their business:

1. Professional liability insurance
2. General liability insurance
3. Property insurance

Professional liability insurance covers you if a client files a lawsuit against you for injuries to him or her as a result of your work, commonly called "malpractice insurance." For years I didn't understand the need for this type of insurance because I was certain I would never harm a client. Then one day I received notice of a lawsuit against me and another massage therapist who worked for me, claiming she had injured a client. Because I owned the business, I was named in the lawsuit as well. The claim ended up being dismissed, thankfully, but I now understand the need for this type of insurance.

General liability insurance covers you if someone is injured on your premises. For example, a client may fall while getting off the massage table or slip on a wet floor. Accidents do happen, and this type of insurance will protect you and your business.

Property insurance protects your premises from events such as a fire or theft. If your business is currently in your home, your homeowner's policy should cover this, but check with your insurance company. Most landlords require this type of insurance from renters.

If you are in need of any or all of the insurance coverage mentioned above, there are several organizations for body workers that offer excellent coverage. Here are some of the popular ones:

- American Massage Council, (800) 500-3930
- American Massage Therapy Association (AMTA), (847) 864-0123
- Associated Bodywork and Massage Professionals (ABMP), (800) 458-2267
- International Massage Association, (540) 351-0800

Two other types of insurance to consider having are disability insurance and health insurance.

Disability insurance will cover loss of income if you become disabled and unable to work. Although not absolutely necessary, you may choose to carry this insurance if you are a one-person business. Once you finish this book and create an equitable business, you probably won't need this type of insurance.

Health insurance covers your healthcare and hospitalization. This is needed by self-employed massage therapists and can be costly. Some massage therapists can obtain coverage under a spouse's insurance plan. If you have employees, you may want to offer this coverage to them. If you are in need of health insurance, look for a group insurance plan for small businesses. Check also with the local chamber of commerce.

BUSINESS CONTRACTS

If you are going to include independent contractors in your business, you will need to prepare a business contract. A business contract is a legally binding promise or set of promises between two parties, such as the owner of the business and the independent contractor (also known as the massage therapist, acupuncturist, or any other professional working within your business). A written business contract spells out the terms of the agreement, and should include:

- The date of the agreement
- Identification of the two parties
- Description of the terms
- Price of consideration
- Signatures of both parties

Questions to ask when preparing your business contract include:

- Who will supply what in the case of linens, oils, table, and so forth?
- Who will pay for liability insurance?
- Are there commissions on product sales?
- Who receives the fees for services?
- What duration will the contract be?

The answers to those questions should be outlined in your business contract.

Once you have prepared your business contract, or at least have answered all of the questions above, consult an attorney to have a legally binding contract prepared. This step is essential to ensure protection for your business. It will eliminate future legal problems, too. A sample business contract is shown in Appendix B, page 73. This sample contract is to be used as a guideline only and does not eliminate the need for you to consult an attorney for your own business contract.

COMPUTERIZING YOUR BUSINESS

You may believe this chapter does not apply to your business, because you've already decided that purchasing a computer, printer, software, Internet service, and paying Web page fees are not within your business budget or even necessary for your business to succeed. If this is how you're feeling that's okay, but promise me you will read this chapter anyway. Once you reach the later chapters of this book, you will better understand just how vital computerizing your business is to maximizing your business success.

Having a computer for your business can serve many functions. It can be used for accounting and recordkeeping purposes, client notetaking records, and preparing business forms such as health intake forms and invoices. More importantly, from a profit standpoint, having a business presence on the Internet can provide basic information about your business, leading to increased income. Ultimately, having a business Web page can allow your clients to schedule appointments even when you're not open for business, get important information about your services, purchase gift certificates and retail products, and more.

The first step is to purchase a computer that will meet your current and future business needs.

Software

Once you have purchased a computer, you can explore software for your business' operational needs. Software programs will help you get organized in your business; however, for the most part they will not directly add profit to your business. Following are suggested companies you may wish to investigate:

- Land Software, 5138 Fulton Street NW, Washington DC 20016, (202) 237-2733, www.landsw.com

- Massageware.com, 5028 First Coast Highway, Fernandina Beach, FL 32034, (800) 520-8514, www.massageware.com

- Island Software Co., 717 Lingco Drive, Richardson, TX 75081, (877) 384-0295, www.islandsoftwareco.com

- Get Physical Software, 15 East Putnam Avenue, Suite 376, Greenwich, CT 06830, (800) 622-0025, www.dancesoft.net

For companies that offer telephone answering services and appointment scheduling, try these:

- Time Trade Systems, Inc., 235 Bear Hill Road, Waltham, MA 02451, (781) 890-4808, www.timetrade.com

- My Receptionist, P.O. Box 0161, 408 Riverside Avenue, Eau Claire, WI 54702, (800) 686-0162, www.my receptionist.com

Internet Presence

Regardless of the size of your business, having business presence on the Internet is a must! It's easy, often free of charge, and doesn't even require you to have a computer; however, you will need access to a computer to input your business information. Many websites offer a free listing for your business; others charge a nominal fee. If you belong to any professional organizations, you can usually list your business free of charge by accessing its website and following the directions.

When listing your business, be sure to provide as much detail about your business as possible. In addition to the business name, address, and telephone number, list your services and training experience, describe the atmosphere of your business, and explain what makes your business exceptional. I added my business to several free websites and within months noticed an increase in business calls, resulting in increased sales.

For listing your business, I recommend you start by looking into these websites, as well as the websites of your member organizations:

- www.massage4life.com
- www.holistic.com
- www.massageresource.com
- www.massagenetwork.com
- www.massageregister.com
- www.onebody.com
- www.massagenet.com

Web Page

Having a Web page for your business is essential for building a successful business. It offers current and prospective clients another convenient means of contacting you. People can view a list of your services, schedule appointments, get directions to your location, and read interesting articles about massage that you post. For the latter, changing the information on a regular basis will encourage return visits to your site. You can sell products and gift certificates 24 hours a day using credit card services. Once built and linked to other Web pages (such as your local chamber of commerce), your business will stand out from many other massage businesses in your area, giving you a leading edge on the market.

You will need to purchase internet service before establishing your business website. Often when purchasing your computer, free internet service, for a limited time, is offered. Many of the popular online services, such as America Online, MSN, and CompuServe offer free introductory trials to try their services. Otherwise, check your local Yellow Pages under "Internet Services" for assistance in setting up service. To create your website, you can either purchase your own software and build your website yourself (if you are computer savvy), or contact a computer college graduate to do it for you, or invest a bit more money and have a professional create one for you. They can be found in the Yellow Pages, under "Website Design Services."

Once you have established your business website, you will need to maintain it by checking it often and updating the information on it. You can also compile email addresses from your clients and send out information to them such as appointment reminders, reminders to purchase holiday gift certificates, and to announce promotions you are offering.

Now it is time to draw business to your website. Begin by informing your clients of your new website by advertising it within your business and mailing either a letter or postcard to them, perhaps with a promotional offer once they enter the website. Second, add your new website address and email address to all marketing materials, such as your business cards, stationery, and Yellow Page ads.

Note that you can track the amount of traffic to your website by adding a counter within the website. This will inform you of the total number of times your website is looked at. It will also help you to determine if your marketing is working.

Part II

Market
Your Business

The methods of marketing you choose for your business will either increase your profits or waste your money. That is why it is essential for you to plan your marketing strategies carefully. Your goal is to find the marketing methods that will give your business the most exposure at the minimal cost to you.

CHAPTER THREE

Marketing

WHAT IS MARKETING ANYWAY?

In simplified terms, marketing is a means of reaching potential clients with information regarding your business. Hopefully, this information will interest the person into utilizing your business to meet his or her needs.

Many massage therapists cringe when it comes to the topic of marketing. There are so many methods of marketing, how do you decide which ones will benefit your business? Will you net a return on your marketing investment or will it be a waste of your hard-earned money? There are endless ways to market your business, some expensive and others free of charge. In this chapter you will learn both no-cost and low-cost methods of marketing, as well as some of the high-cost methods of marketing to avoid.

NO-COST MARKETING

When I hear the phrase "no cost," I immediately think of the television advertisements where the obnoxious car salesman, standing in the middle of a car lot, offers "no money down and cash back" deals on new cars. No-cost marketing is similar in that you don't pay any money for the marketing and hope you will receive "cash back" with increased business. Although these no-cost methods of marketing will not cost you any money, some will cost you time. Here are some "risk-free" methods.

Word of mouth. This method is the number one way to market your business. Here's how it works. One of your satisfied clients leaves your business, tells another person how wonderful your business is, and the other person tries your business. I make it a habit to tell a client who asks me if I accept tips (gratuities) that the best tip they can give me is a referral. Don't be afraid to ask your clients if they know someone who can benefit from your services. Tell everyone you meet about your business. Become comfortable talking about massage to new people you meet. Remember, every person you meet is a potential new client, so spread the word.

Tip: After a new client pays me for their treatment, I will say, "Would you like to schedule another massage or would you like to take my business card and call for a future appointment?" In doing this, the client isn't put on the spot to make another appointment and he or she leaves my office with a business card in hand.

Press releases. A press release is a typewritten announcement sent to local newspapers that gives information about your business—perhaps your business opening, advanced training you've taken, a new professional who has joined your business, new services you're offering, and so forth. Send out press releases every time a positive event occurs within your business. Make certain your press releases are typewritten, double-spaced, and the envelope and top of the press release read "For Immediate Release." Your name and telephone number are typed at the bottom of the press release. A sample press release is in Appendix B, page 76.

Lectures. Call your local business associations (for instance, the Knights of Columbus and Elks Lodge) and offer to do a presentation about the benefits of massage, reflexology, or any other related topic. Most associations have weekly lunch meetings for members and are always looking for meeting topics. Once you give your lecture, pass around your business cards and brochures, and make sure to bring your appointment book with you. You can also offer a five-minute chair massage demonstration to entice members into scheduling an appointment with you on the spot.

Answering machine or voicemail. Your answering machine or voicemail can be used for more than taking messages while you're not available. A friendly message, full of pertinent information, may very well answer callers' questions. My business message was as follows: "Thank you for calling Professional Massage Associates. Today is Monday, March 15th. We are open and we do have appointments available for today; however, we are currently with clients at this time. If you would like information regarding office hours and directions, press 1; for information regarding our services and rates, press 2; or you may leave a message after the tone and we will call you back shortly. Thank you."

After pressing 1, the message was, "We are conveniently located at 7 Wells Street in Saratoga Springs. From the north end of Broadway at the Sheraton Hotel, turn left onto Van Dam Street; go six blocks and turn right onto Wells Street. We are the third building on the left. Our office hours are Monday through Friday, 9 A.M. to 7 P.M., and Saturdays 9 A.M. to 2 P.M. If you would like to leave a message now, we will call you back shortly. Thank you."

After pressing 2, the message was, "Our services include professional massages at $35 per half hour and $55 per hour; foot reflexology treatments at $55 for one hour; cranio-sacral therapy at $65 for 75 minutes; hot stone massage at $75 for one hour and $100 for 90 minutes; European facials at $55; Chinese herbal consultations at $50; and acupuncture treatments at $60 each. We offer gift certificates and accept MasterCard and Visa. If you would like to leave a message now, we will call you back shortly. Thank you."

Many basic telephone answering machines and voicemail services offer mailbox features that you can use to deliver information such as the messages above. Also note that I stated the current date at the beginning of the message (which I naturally changed every day) because it immediately told the caller that we were open, checking messages, and had appointments available that day. This is what a large number of callers want to know, but when they get a basic answering machine message, they tend to hang up and try another listing. I immediately noticed an increase in messages when I added the current date. Try it!

Networking with physicians. Send a letter to local physicians, such as chiropractors, general practitioners, orthopedists, and dentists, announcing your business and services. (A sample letter is in Appendix B, page 77.) Follow up on the letter by visiting the physician's office and introducing yourself to both the physician and staff. You may want to take a binder with photographs of your business and present them to the physicians so they have an idea of what the business looks like. Perhaps you can offer the physician a courtesy 30-minute massage certificate to try your services.

If you accept insurance reimbursement, make mention of this in your letter. Then when you visit the physician, bring along a referral pad to leave with the physician. (A sample is shown in Appendix B, page 80.) It is also good business etiquette to send a handwritten "thank you" for all referrals.

Email clients. If you have a computer with Internet services, you can send your clients occasional notices regarding specials you are offering, new services and products, and holiday gift certificate reminders (as well as appointment confirmations). First, compile a list of your clients who have email addresses. Then, approximately once a month, send them an email. This omits the cost of printing, envelopes, and stamps. It may take an hour of your time to prepare the email, but it won't cost anything to send it. You could also send the same message you chose for your in-office displays (mentioned later).

Chair massage demonstration. This is a popular way to promote your business and educate people about your services. Because massage is a personal service, many people feel more comfortable meeting their therapist in advance and receiving a clothed massage. Although a professional massage chair is optimal, you can use a regular chair and tabletop instead, or even rent a chair from another massage therapist for the day.

Look for busy, high-volume places to do chair massage demonstrations, such as shopping malls, store grand openings, health fairs, college events, or sporting events. Offer complimentary 5- or 10-minute massages. Bring your business cards, brochures, gift certificates, appointment book, short health intake forms (use the addresses for future mailings), photographs of your business, disposable face cradle covers, and sanitation wipes for cleansing between treatments. It is also important to dress professionally and wear a name tag.

The optimal time to offer chair massage demonstrations in shopping malls is during peak holiday shopping times, such as Christmas and Valentine's Day, because you can sell a lot of gift certificates to stressed-out people. It's the perfect "one size fits all" gift.

LOW-COST MARKETING

After you have tried some or all of the no-cost marketing methods outlined above, utilize some of these low-cost marketing methods. By doing so, you incur a minimal cost and a small risk on your investment.

Business cards. A good business card is the number one low-cost marketing method. Have about 500 to 1,000 cards printed. Make certain your name, credentials, address, telephone number, and website address are included and spelled correctly. Some therapists use double-sided cards with appointment information printed on the reverse side. It is important that your cards be professional and of good quality. Business cards printed off of computers on flimsy paper do not portray a professional image, although there is better quality paper stock available these days for computer printing. It is also not very professional to have information on your card crossed out and changed with ink. When information on your card changes, please get new cards.

Always carry your business cards with you. Hand them out everywhere you go. Make certain your hairdresser, nail technician, physician, and any other person you do business with has some of your cards on hand to pass out for you. In return, keep their business cards for cross-referring. It always pleases me to sit in my hairdresser's chair and see my business cards displayed nearby.

Your business cards can also be displayed on bulletin boards locally, perhaps at the health food store, exercise facilities, and coffee shops. Look around for free bulletin boards.

Brochures. A brochure is a source of information regarding your business. It lists your fees along with a description of each service. Additional information also included would be methods of payment, such as credit cards, hours of operation, "gift certificates available," product lines you carry, a map or directions to your location, and of course your name, address, telephone number, and website address.

Once again, it is important your brochures be professional and of good quality. Brochures printed off the computer on regular copy-quality paper do not portray a professional image. However, you can purchase thicker quality stock paper for computer printing, or use a printing company.

Some therapists purchase professional brochures featuring certain topics about massage, foot reflexology, sports massage, and so forth. If you purchase professional brochures, adhere a sticker with your business name, address, telephone number, and website address to the back of the brochure for contact information.

Some companies that offer professional brochures include:

- Hemingway Publications, Inc., (815) 877-5590, www.hemingwaymassageproducts.com
- Information for People, (800) 754-9790, www.info4people. com.

Once your brochure is ready, distribute it locally to hotels (if there is a concierge, introduce yourself), bed and breakfasts, coffee shops, and businesses with which you do business. Check frequently to see if more brochures are needed, especially in the hotels.

Display your brochure in your reception area and offer to mail it to potential clients making inquiries on the telephone. I also attach a brochure to each gift certificate that has a gift of a dollar amount, rather than a specific service, on it. That way, the recipient can choose the services they would like.

In-office displays. The reception area, bathroom, and each treatment room are excellent locations to place an attractive display ad in a picture frame. Here you can advertise new or current services, holiday gift certificate reminders, retail products, and promotions. For my business, I made the color displays myself on the computer and changed them monthly. For example, as the weather became colder, I placed a display that read, "Warm up with a hot stone massage." This display sparked my clients to inquire about the service, leading to my scheduling appointments. Our office used a special pregnancy pillow for prenatal massages, and whenever I displayed the ad, many clients would comment that they didn't know you could receive a massage during pregnancy. After educating them, I would recommend they purchase a gift certificate for any expectant mothers they knew. In-office displays are great reminders for gift certificates, especially at Christmastime, Valentine's Day, and Mother's Day. When we began offering European facials, we offered a free eyebrow wax with each one-hour facial. We also placed a brochure, explaining each type of facial treatment, next to the display ad. Our facial appointments increased!

Newsletters. Mailing periodic newsletters to existing clientele and prospective clients is another effective method of educating people on the many benefits your services provide, as well as announcing new services, products, and promotions, and simply keeping connected to your clients. Each time a newsletter is received by a client, it serves as a reminder to make an appointment or purchase a gift certificate.

You can create your own newsletters tailored specifically to your business, or you can purchase professional newsletters typeset with your business name. Your own creative newsletters will take time to prepare and print, but the benefit of doing so is that they are more personalized and you control all of the information on them. You can purchase professional newsletters from companies such as Staying in Touch, (877) 634-1010, www.stayingintouch.net. This company allows you to add some personalized information to the standard newsletter.

Refer a friend. Some therapists offer discounts for their services, such as "buy one, get one free." I believe this is way too much of a discount and may rebut your professional image. I recommend offering a referral program with your existing clients. Tell existing clients that you are striving to build your business and would appreciate their help. Ask them to recommend you to their friends, family, and business associates, and offer in return to take $5 off your client's next visit for each referral. Or you can offer them 15 extra minutes on their next visit. (Note: This offer does not apply to gift certificate purchases.) Make this an ongoing offer, without expiration. Just think, it will cost you a marketing investment of only $5.00 (or 15 minutes of your time) to obtain a new client. It's a win-win situation. You get a new client and your existing client receives a discount of $5 (or an additional 15 minutes) on their next visit. You may want to take this marketing method even further by placing this offer in a display sign in your office, and/or announcing it in your newsletters or emails.

Networking organizations. A great way to market your business is by joining local business organizations such as the chamber of commerce or networking groups. There is usually an annual membership fee but there are benefits that come with it. Keep in mind, however, that you will need to partake in the activities such as business networking "mixers" and meetings to benefit from this method of marketing. You might want to attend an event first before investing your money. Often, the chamber of commerce will have networking "mixers" at a local establishment where you can pay a small fee of perhaps $5 to $20 to mingle with other business professionals while passing out your business cards.

Telephone directory (Yellow Pages). I highly recommend having your business listed in your local telephone directory. But watch out because it can be expensive if you are not careful about the size of your advertisement. Listing your business in the telephone directory is essential for capturing those out-of-town guests thumbing through the Yellow Pages. It's also beneficial for new residents and convenient for existing clientele.

The size of your listing will depend on the amount of competitive businesses already listed under the massage category. If there are only a few listings, you can keep your listing small, perhaps with a bold, all-capital letter listing or an in-column display ad, featuring information about your business. This way, your business will stand out from the others. If, however, there are many listings, it may be beneficial to add color to your listing. But again, be aware of extra costs. (A sample ad is shown in Appendix B, page 81.)

If you decide to invest in a display ad, you will need to make it appealing to the consumer. Use words that describe the benefits of your services such as "reduce stress, relieve pain, heal, and relax." List the services you offer, mention that gift certificates are available, and specify which methods of payment you accept. Naturally, your business name, address, telephone number, and website will be listed.

As mentioned earlier, if you are just beginning your business, choose a business name that starts with the beginning of the alphabet (A, B, C) because it will be listed first, increasing your chances of being called first.

HIGH-COST MARKETING

If you have been in the massage business for any length of time, you have been approached by many advertising companies trying to lure you into expensive marketing campaigns that usually net you few dollars. The display ads can be very attractive; however, they may not hit your target market. Often they are so expensive, it is unlikely you will net a return on your investment.

What is a target market anyway? A target market reaches the specific people who will likely use your services. For example, if you specialize in sports massage, your target market would be athletes, local sporting stores, health clubs, and orthopedic physicians. If you specialize in prenatal massage, your target market would be expectant mothers, birth instructors, local baby clothing stores, and obstetric physicians. You need to determine what your target market is and place your advertisements in those specific areas where your target clientele will see them.

Here are some examples of high-cost marketing methods.

Radio advertisements. If your business is a large day spa and it is approaching Valentine's Day, this means of marketing might pay off. However, it's very difficult to sell your business via the radio. Most people are doing other things while listening to the radio, such as driving a car, and can't even write down your telephone number. It will take numerous radio ads before your message will start to become effective. Also, it is very difficult to determine how many new clients you actually obtain from this means of marketing.

Television advertisements. Again, the ads are pricey and the return on investment is unpredictable.

Newspaper advertising. If you are tempted to try newspaper advertising, use small ads and repeat the ad frequently, rather than using one large ad. Newspaper advertising can be beneficial for selling gift certificates at peak holiday times but don't get roped into an expensive ad that is surrounded by 50 other advertisements. If you do decide to use newspaper advertising, ask the salesperson if the paper will do a free story on your business if you advertise with them. Newspapers need stories, and you might just get some free public relations out of it!

ADVERTISING COMPARISONS

Let's compare some of the different types of advertising:

- Newspaper—reaches a large audience in a specific region but has a short life span because people throw it out quickly.

- Magazine—reaches a large audience in a specific target market and has a long life span because people tend to retain it and circulate it.

- Telephone directory—reaches a large audience looking for your services, advertising payments are made by monthly installments, gives information regarding your business, and listings are alphabetical.

- Direct mail—reaches a target market inexpensively and is likely to have a long life span because it is retained by the receiver.

CHAPTER FOUR

Additional Income

GIFT CERTIFICATES

Offering gift certificates for sale in your business is the single most profitable business decision you can make. It astonishes me when I hear massage therapists say they don't bother with selling gift certificates. They are your very best referral system. In other words, each redeemed gift certificate by a new client is free advertising for you because you didn't have to pay for the referral. In addition, each time a new client redeems a gift certificate, you have the opportunity to make him or her a client. He or she is also more inclined to purchase another gift certificate for someone else and/or purchase products from you.

There are more great reasons for selling gift certificates. A percentage of recipients never redeem the gift certificate. In this case, you earn money for doing nothing.

Selling gift certificates will increase your cash flow! Some therapists don't like this feature because they spend the money and then feel like they are doing a "free" massage when the recipient finally comes in for the appointment. I have never understood this complaint. If someone wants to pay me money in advance for a service—that, by the way, I may never have to perform—I'm all for it!

Six Ways to Increase Gift Certificate Sales

1. Produce high quality, attractive gift certificates. Self-made paper gift certificates are not desirable. Remember, these are "gift" certificates. You can either have a specially designed gift certificate printed for your business by your local printer, or you can purchase bulk gift certificates. Try one of the following places:
   - Hemingway Publications (815) 877-5590, www.hemingwaymassageproducts.com
   - Information For People, (800) 754-9790, www.info4people.com

2. Package your gift certificates for an event or holiday. For Christmas, place each gift certificate in an elegant box and attach a bow to it. For Valentine's Day, place each gift certificate in a red box and attach a chocolate heart-shaped lollipop to the box with a ribbon. For other events, such as birthdays, place each gift certificate in a small gift bag, stuffed with tissue and confetti. Display these gift certificate creations throughout your business so clients can see them.

    You can also create gift baskets, full of products and a gift certificate, for the ultimate gift. For example, you can combine massage oil, aroma scents, a scented candle, and a gift certificate into a small basket and wrap it with clear cellophane and a red ribbon. Display gift baskets in your reception area.

3. Make use of display advertising within your business. Place a "Gift Certificates Available" sign in a picture frame in each treatment room, the reception area, and the bathroom. The more the client sees this reminder, the more gift certificates you will sell. Also, as clients check out, ask if they need a gift certificate for anyone special.

4. Advertise "gift certificates available" on all marketing materials, including brochures, Yellow Pages ads, newsletters, Web page, and so forth. Also make certain your answering machine message mentions gift certificates.

5. Network with other businesses who will sell your gift certificates for you for a percentage. For example, give ten gift

certificates and a display ad to your personal trainer, hairdresser, nail technician, or other business owner, and offer them $10 to $15 for each gift certificate they sell. Remember, not all gift certificates are redeemed. If no gift certificates are sold, you haven't incurred any costs in advertising. If gift certificates are sold, you pay $10 or $15 for each new client. (Instead of a percentage, you can barter services with the professional—for instance, a one-hour massage for every four gift certificates sold.)

Find a florist who will sell your gift certificates during peak holidays, such as Valentine's Day, Mother's Day, and Secretaries Day. Have the florist attach your gift certificate to the card holder fork and display it at the shop. This will enhance the gift.

6. Wholesale your gift certificates to businesses that give gifts to customers and employees. Realtors, car salespeople, and small business firms often "thank" their customers and employees with gifts. Sell 10 one-hour massage gift certificates for $375. Make sure the gift certificates are given only as gifts and are nontransferable, and place a one-year expiration date on them. Again, remember that not all gift certificates are redeemed.

Find a bed-and-breakfast owner who will purchase one gift certificate for each guest to add to a Valentine's Day overnight package. You might even choose to go to the bed and breakfast and spend the day working there. This may even turn into a regular event. Satisfied guests will tell the owner, and you may get many more referrals.

EDUCATIONAL CLASSES

Holding classes is a great way to increase your income. Other than time, there is no cost to you and there are many benefits. By educating people about massage and other services, you increase your odds of obtaining them as clients. Some good places to hold classes are at your local high school where continuing education classes are periodically offered, or at your own business if you have enough room. You can teach a one-day class or a series of classes, perhaps one class on massage techniques, another on foot reflexology, and another on aromatherapy.

While teaching your students about massage use retail products you sell, such as massage oils, candles, aromatherapy oils, music, books, hand tools, herbal eye pillows, and so forth. Display these items on a table and at the end of each class sell them. You can also sell gift certificates and make appointments. You may even offer a small discount to students who schedule an appointment or purchase a gift certificate at the end of class. Make sure to bring along photos of your business, your appointment book, business cards, and brochures. Set the atmosphere with soothing music, aroma, and low lighting.

If your business consists of more than one therapist, teach a series of classes and have each therapist choose a different topic to teach at each class. This way, the students get to meet every therapist.

Part III

Build Equity

Now that you have established your business and used the marketing methods listed in the previous chapters to build clientele, it is time to build equity in your business. Building equity in your business adds value to it, which will give you a return of income when you decide to retire, relocate, or change careers. After all, don't you deserve to receive compensation for your years of hard work?

CHAPTER FIVE

How to Build Equity

Many massage therapists work for several years only to walk away from their business because it has no equity and cannot be sold. Think about your current massage business. Would anyone purchase your business from you right now if you listed it for sale? If so, what would they be buying? If all you have to sell is your clientele, you will have a difficult time selling your client list for more than a few hundred dollars, because there is no guarantee any of your clients will become clients of the new list owner.

This chapter will give you the needed tools to build equity in your business, even if the business is located in your home. It is more challenging to sell a home-based business, but it is certainly possible. (Chapter 6 gives you more information regarding a home-based business.)

SERVICES

Offering massage therapy services is often the only service massage therapists have to offer to their clients. The client comes to your business, receives a massage treatment, and leaves. The client will then refer to other businesses for a variety of different types of services.

In order to build equity in your business, you need to offer your clients an array of services. You can start by adding different types of massage treatments such as shiatsu, neuromuscular therapy,

44

myofascial release, lymphatic drainage, prenatal, aromatherapy, cranio-sacral therapy, hot stone massage, and foot reflexology. All of these services complement the Swedish massage, yet offer other methods of treatment for your clients to choose from. This will give you a competitive edge.

If your business leans more toward pampering or relaxing services, you could add services such as facials, manicures/pedicures, paraffin treatments, body wraps, hydrotherapy (baths), steam, sauna, and electrolysis or waxing. These added services will increase your revenue and add value to your business. Why refer your client elsewhere for these services, when you can offer them at your business? Clients like the convenience of going to one business to receive multiple services.

If your business leans more toward medical massage or has a clinical atmosphere, you could add services such as acupuncture, herbal medicine, chiropractic, nutritional counseling, and stretching and/or yoga instruction. These added services will also increase your revenue and add value to your business. Your clients will appreciate the convenience of multiple services at one location.

The idea in adding services to your business is not for you to perform them all; this would not help you build equity in your business. Besides, you would need additional training and licenses for some of the added services. Although you can learn a variety of massage treatments to add to your credentials, to build business equity, you will need to add staff to your business.

INDEPENDENT CONTRACTORS

Another way to build equity in your business is to earn money while you're not working. Yes, you've read that sentence right. In order to do this, you need to add independent contractors to your business. This is the key to building equity and having a business you can sell. And nothing is more rewarding than to know that while you are not working, you are earning income. By adding independent contractors to my business, I increased my annual income by more than $30,000.

After deciding what new services to add to your business, seek the professionals who will perform these services. You can place an advertisement in the classified section of your local newspaper, call schools who train the professionals, or ask around for a referral.

It is important the person or persons you contract with for services share the same business values and ideas you do. Ask them what their long-term goals are because you do not want to contract with someone whose intention is to build a business under your roof and then open their own business down the street from you.

Independent contractors differ from employees, and I highly recommend you contract with professionals instead of hiring employees. Hiring employees entails payroll, employee taxes, and social security benefits—the paperwork can overwhelm you. On the other hand, independent contractors are responsible for their own taxes, and your only work involves signing a business agreement with each other. (A sample business contract is shown in Appendix B, page 73.)

Having independent contractors in your business instead of employees does, however, give you less control of some decisions. For example, you cannot mandate what attire independent contractors wear or set their work schedule. (A sample comparison is shown in Appendix A, page 72.) Nonetheless, adding independent contractors to your business is easier than having employees.

As you add each new independent contractor to your business, make the appropriate announcements to your clients and to the public. Refer back to the marketing chapters to promote the new services. Then, watch your business grow even more.

RETAIL PRODUCTS

The third step in building equity in your business is to add retail products. Some massage therapists feel like they would be "pushing" retail on their clients and refuse to carry any retail products. You are doing your clients a disservice by not carrying retail products and you are doing your business a disservice by limiting your income.

How often does a client ask you during their treatment what oil or lotion you are using or comment on the scent of aromatherapy they are smelling? Do you ever suggest your clients purchase a product to help with or prevent pain? Wouldn't it be convenient if your client could obtain these products right at your business?

It is not necessary to "push" products in order to sell them. You simply need to use them in your treatments. They will sell themselves. Adding retail products to your business can add thousands of dollars per month to your income. It also makes your business more sellable because it is another means of income for the business.

Here are some examples of products your business could sell: massage oils/lotions, candles, aromatherapy scents, relaxation music, bath products, skin and body care products (if you offer facial and/or body treatments), hot and cold packs, herbal eye pillows, heatable rice bags, cervical pillows, massage and/or relaxation videos, lumbar supports, magnetic therapy products, and any other products you use in your business or recommend to clients.

Check for product advertisements in local massage magazines and call your professional suppliers to inquire about wholesale product service. If your state collects sales tax on merchandise, you will also need to obtain a state sales tax certificate before selling retail. This certificate can be obtained by calling your state sales tax office.

Once you have decided on which retail products to carry, you will need to display them for clients to see and touch. The reception area is the best location for retail. Clients can shop while waiting for their appointment. Make sure the clients can reach the products to handle them, otherwise they won't purchase them. If there are sample sizes available, place them in front of the retail products and mark them "tester" so clients can try them. Be sure to clearly mark the retail price on the bottom of the product.

Next, educate your staff about the products and offer them a small percentage of income for each product they sell—maybe 10 or 15 percent. This will help you to sell even more retail, while giving your staff an incentive to sell.

Again, remember that you need to use the products in your treatments or recommend them if you are going to sell them.

TIME AND SPACE

Efficient use of time and space in your business is another key to increasing your income. Since you can only physically work so many hours per day, per week, why not maximize the usage of each treatment room so it is being used all day long? For example, if you start your day at 9:00 A.M. and perform five massages, finishing your day at 3:30 P.M., instead of turning the lights out and closing your business, why not have another professional use the room for treatments from 4:00 until 9:00 P.M.? By doing this, you will expand your business hours, the professional will earn income, and you will earn income from their rent to you. Furthermore, the professional has the opportunity to sell retail or a gift certificate, earning you even more income. This is called efficient usage of time.

The ultimate goal is to utilize each treatment room 80 to 85 percent of the time (since 100 percent is nearly impossible) seven days per week. In addition, if you, the owner, choose not to work on weekends, contract with other professionals to work during those times as well. With a 12-hour per day schedule, you can split shifts between two professionals per room, so each professional can work a full day.

Efficient usage of space means you can perform a variety of treatments in each room. Hence, one room isn't dedicated to just one treatment. For example, a facial room can also be a massage room if you have a versatile table that folds in the middle and can be adjusted into a chair. A facial or massage room also can double as a wet room for water treatments if you have a drain in the floor and an area rug placed over it when doing a massage. Hydrotherapy tubs also come with massage table tops as an option. Making each treatment room versatile will make it easier to maximize the number of appointments in each room.

STEP OUTSIDE THE BOX

You've probably heard this phrase—it's one of my favorites. Inside the "box" is where most people remain, offering the usual standard services and customer service to their clients. When you step outside the box, you do something unusual and unique that makes your clients feel special and catches them off guard. Adjusting your customer service level to offer exceptional service will bring them back to you over and over again.

So how do you step outside the box? The first step is to take a few minutes to answer these questions. Really think about each question and write down your answers before continuing:

- What can I do differently to make my clients feel cared for?
- How can I surprise my clients with a kind gesture?
- What standard services can I make exceptional for my clients that my competitors do not offer?

Did you come up with some good answers? If you didn't yet answer the questions, please stop now and go back and answer them.

One example of stepping outside the box and offering outstanding customer service is to offer to deliver gift certificates to clients as a complimentary service. Offering to deliver gift certificates is a really nice service your customers will greatly appreciate, and they will think of you when they need a last-minute gift and have no time for shopping. Try advertising this service and see how well it works. This is especially good to promote during the busy holidays.

Another example is to send your most loyal clients a birthday card on their birthday, with a personalized, handwritten note telling them that you value them. Think of what a surprise that will be to your client. It's a simple, kind gesture that will mean a lot.

If your client is coming in on his or her birthday, have a gourmet cupcake with a candle in it waiting for them. What a great surprise! It is said that 80 percent of your business is done by 20 percent of your clients. Make sure you are taking care of them.

One business I always think of as an example of stepping outside the box is an Italian restaurant in Baltimore. They offer complimentary limousine transportation to and from their establishment. The limousine drives all over the city, with its advertisement on the vehicle, transporting happy customers. The customers are more apt to drink more if they don't have to drive home. It's also convenient for out-of-town visitors who do not know the area well because they don't have to worry about getting lost. This is an exceptional, unique service.

If you are looking for a good book to inspire you, read *If It Ain't Broke, Break It* by Dr. Robert Kriegel.

MINIMIZE OVERHEAD

Every business has expenses. Some are set expenses, such as rent and monthly Yellow Page advertising costs, and some are variable expenses you have every month but the amount fluctuates. If you want to build equity in your business, it is important to know what your expenses are and to minimize them whenever possible. Your business will have greater value if your income is high and your expenses are low. It also exemplifies good business management.

The largest expense is usually your rent. This is a great place to work on minimizing your overhead. Before you sign a lease, explore ways of negotiating a better deal. For example, before I signed another three-year lease with my landlord, I asked other tenants what they were paying per square foot for their rented space. I then shopped around to other locations in town and found a vacant space with the same square footage I had, but it was $3 per square foot less than my new lease would be. I really didn't want to move, but I thought if I had the lesser lease in hand, it would be a good negotiating tool for lowering my new lease. It worked! My landlord reduced the new lease by $3 per square foot and I saved $9,000 in overhead over a three-year period. I can't guarantee this will work for you, but it is certainly worth trying.

The next place to minimize your overhead is with your linen service (if you have one). In my region, I learned I didn't have to sign a contract with a linen vendor in order to get service. They, of course, pressed me to sign a contract but were willing to service me when I said no. This left me with flexibility to negotiate a better price or find another vendor. I called other massage therapists in town and found the prices they paid for linens varied, and I was paying more than others with the same vendor. I then called competitive linen vendors and researched their prices. My final call was to my existing linen vendor—whose service I really liked—and insisted they match the lower prices. They did! I saved my business more than $100 per month just by making a few phone calls.

These are just two examples of ways to minimize your overhead. You can also reduce your expenses for your telephone service, including long distance service, credit card merchant fees, and bank account fees. Take a look at your monthly bills and then start working on reducing your overhead.

The 10 Steps to Success

If you have read this book from the beginning, you are now ready to apply the information you have learned. Here are the 10 steps that will lead you to a successful business, built with equity:

1. Give outstanding customer service
2. Increase gift certificate sales
3. Give educational classes
4. Utilize the marketing methods listed in this book
5. Add more services to your menu
6. Add independent contractors to your business
7. Make efficient use of time and space in each treatment room
8. Sell retail products
9. Offer credit cards as a method of payment
10. Decrease business expenses (overhead) wherever possible

CHAPTER SIX

Home-Based Business

WORKING FROM HOME

Some massage therapists choose to run their business out of a dedicated area of their home. The business often consists of a treatment room, a waiting area, and access to a bathroom. If this sounds like your massage therapy business, this chapter is important for you to read.

By now, if you've read this book in its entirety, you've learned how to establish your business, how to market it, and how to build equity in it. But because your business is located within your home, you are probably wondering how you are going to sell it when the time comes. First, let me assure you that it is possible to sell a home-based business; however, there are some additional steps to take to accomplish this.

The first step for you is to build up your retail and gift certificate sales. This will make your business more valuable and show a prospective buyer that the business generates income other than your hands-on work.

The next step has to do with the services you offer. If you add a few more types of massage, you will increase your credentials, however, in the long run it will be difficult to find a buyer who will have your same credentials, who can offer the same treatments to your clients. Therefore, it is essential that you add at least one independent contractor to your business. This will increase your business' value. If you have only one treatment room, you can split shifts and maximize the use of the room. If your massage schedule is full, you can offer the independent contractor all "overflow" clients as an incentive for him or her to work out of your home. If the independent contractor offers different services than you, you can refer your own clients to him or her.

If you find it impossible to contract with an independent contractor who is willing to work out of your home-based business, you will need to find a place to relocate your business. Remember, this will only be temporary for you, to help you prepare the business for sale. You should do this between one and two years before you plan to sell the business. This will ease your clients into a new location, while maintaining you as their therapist.

I would advise you to not tell your clients your intention of selling the business. You don't want to instill fear in them and have them start looking for a new therapist. I would also advise you to not share your future intentions of selling your business with any of your independent contractors to ensure that word doesn't spread. Who knows, when the time comes, one of them may purchase your business.

These steps will put you on track for the successful sale of your business.

Part IV

Profit From Your Business

By now you have put tremendous amounts of time, energy, and hard work into your business. You have completed the first three stages of this book by (1) establishing your business, (2) marketing it successfully, and (3) building equity and value in the business. Now you can begin thinking about the final stage of getting out of your business and making a profit.

CHAPTER SEVEN

Capitalize On
Your Business

You may not be ready for this stage right now, but at some point you will be asking yourself what's the best way to untangle yourself from the business you've dedicated so much time into putting together. Or you may be ready for this final stage because you are looking forward to retiring to some beautiful, warm climate. Or you may be looking to relocate for personal or health reasons. Perhaps you are simply tired of the massage business and looking for a way out. Regardless of your reasons, it is important you not wait until one of these events hits you over the head. Begin thinking about your strategy now, even if you are years away from selling your business. This way, you will have sufficient time to put your plan in place, therefore optimizing your chances of successfully selling your business for the highest price. If you wait until you need to sell the business, you may significantly decrease your options and profits.

It took me two years to sell my massage therapy business. I tried unsuccessfully for one year to sell it myself. Although I had some offers during that time, they were for about 50 percent of my offering price, and I was willing to wait for a better offer. After one year, I hired a business broker to sell the business for me. He told me it would take one year, and it did, but I sold the business for exactly the price I thought it was worth. Although two years seemed like a long time, looking back now, I feel my patience paid off. Through this experience, I gained a lot of knowledge on the "art" of selling a massage therapy business.

There are a few options to choose from once you decide to get out of your business. You can either (1) liquidate your business and sell your client list, or (2) sell your business. Another option would be to simply close your business and walk away; however, after all your hard work, that is hardly a smart choice. Planning now for this event will eliminate your having to make the last choice.

LIQUIDATE YOUR ASSETS

Liquidating your assets means selling all of the tangible business items for as much money as you can get. If your business has no real value other than the assets, you will need to liquidate them instead of selling the business. This is why building equity in your business is absolutely essential. It builds value!

If you choose to liquidate your business instead of selling it, you will net considerably less money from the sale. If time is of the essence, you may want to go this route for it is usually much quicker to liquidate your business than it is to sell it. Some massage therapists need to relocate quickly for health or personal reasons. This being the case, liquidating your business will make sense.

In order to liquidate your business, you will first need to make a complete list of all of the business assets. This includes all equipment, furnishings, and supplies. This process involves writing down each item you see in every room of your business. Then assign a fair market value to each item. The fair market value will be the price you believe the item is worth. The value is typically less than what it cost new (unless the item has appreciated), but more than you would sell it for in a garage sale. The condition of each item will also determine the value. It is helpful to know the original cost of each item. When your list is complete, type up a master list of all items with their assigned values. You may wish to group together your smaller items, such as office supplies and music, and sell them together.

Next, you will need to prepare a mailing list of all persons and businesses you believe may be interested in purchasing your assets. Make sure to include the massage therapists in your local area and other like businesses. Massage therapy schools are also great places to market. New graduating students may be looking for items to outfit their new offices.

Prepare a flyer to distribute to your prospective buyers and mail it out. You may want to attach your complete list of items for sale or just mention a few of the larger items. You can also place an advertisement in your local newspaper(s), announcing the liquidation sale. If you do this, I recommend you set a specific date and time for prospective buyers to view the items. This will save you the hassle of walk-ins at inconvenient times.

As you sell each item, mark down on paper who you sold the item to and for how much money. Be prepared to give each buyer a receipt for purchase. To do this, you can make up an invoice on the computer or purchase a receipt book at an office supply store.

SELL YOUR CLIENT LIST

If you have decided to liquidate your business, you can also sell your client list to one of your colleagues or to a similar business. Your client list will consist of the names and current addresses of all of your clients, as well as the frequency of their business. For confidentiality reasons you should not sell your client files without the permission of each client. If your client requests their file be transferred to the purchaser of your client list (or any other professional), make a copy of the file and give it directly to the client to make the transfer. This will eliminate any legal issues.

In order to sell your client list, you will need to sign a "covenant not to compete" clause. This clause, in general, states that upon the sale of your client list you agree to not contact the clients for business. In addition, you agree to not open up a massage therapy business within a certain radius of your current business for a specific number of years. This noncompete clause protects the buyer from your soliciting the clients for business after the client list is sold. It is important to have a business attorney create this document for you, but wait until you have a buyer before investing the money. Without this document, your client list has no value.

Purchasing a client list is risky to the purchaser because there is no guarantee the clients will become new clients for the purchaser of the list. You can, however, reduce the risk somewhat by offering to recommend your clients to the purchaser, perhaps by sending a letter to each of your clients. Still, there is no guarantee.

Your client list is worth as much as someone is willing to pay. Therefore, you will need to determine an offering price and negotiate from there. To determine the value of your client list, divide it into three categories: regular clients, occasional clients, and one-time clients. Regular clients are those who frequent your business within every two months. Occasional clients visit your business infrequently, on more of an as-needed basis. One-time clients have visited your business only one, maybe two times. Your regular clients will have a greater value than the occasional clients, and the occasional clients will have a greater value than the one-time clients.

Now that you have established three lists of clients, you will need to attach a dollar amount to each category to be multiplied by the total number of clients in each category. Ask yourself what it will be worth to the purchaser to receive one of your regular clients as their new client? If Jane comes to your business every two weeks, producing a gross annual income to your business of $1,400, what value can you place on that new business? Conversely, how valuable is an occasional client to the purchaser? Finally, how valuable is a list of clients who have visited your business only one or two times? You will need to place a value for each type of client, which can be very subjective.

Here is an example of a client list with assigned values:

Client List		Dollar Value	Total
Regular clients: 50	x	$55	$2,750
Occasional clients: 100	x	$25	$2,500
One-time clients: 200	x	$15	$3,000
Total client list value:			$8,250

Using this calculation, your total client list value is $8,250. For negotiating purposes, I would recommend your offering price for selling your client list be $10,500. This will leave you with $2,250 to negotiate with. Once you have determined your offering price, decide what your bottom-line offer will be. In other words, what is the least amount of money you are willing to accept for the sale of your client list? Perhaps in this example your bottom-line offer would be $6,000. Now you are prepared to negotiate any offers for your client list.

The longer you have been in business, the more likely your client list will be larger. Remember, however, that your one-time client list may have clients whom you haven't seen in many years and their address information may have changed, so the value of your one-time clients may be even lower if you cannot verify the correct addresses of those clients.

As a word of caution, be very discreet and selective when choosing to approach prospective buyers of your client list. It would be disappointing to say the least if a prospective buyer chose not to purchase your client list and then moved into your leased space after you closed your doors. They would reap the benefits of your clients without paying you for the referrals. Sadly, I have seen this happen. Situation: The owner of the client list doesn't sell the client list, and instead ends up closing the business. A prospective buyer of the client list then leases the space and opens a massage business. The clients on the list remain at the familiar location and the owner of the new business gets the clients without paying for the client list. It's best not to mention when you are vacating your leased space. Instead, mention that you have other prospective buyers interested in purchasing your client list, without disclosing any names.

CHAPTER EIGHT

Sell Your Business

When I began my massage therapy career in 1991, selling a massage therapy practice was practically unheard of. Today, I see advertisements in almost every journal and on numerous massage websites. The massage therapy field has increased dramatically, and many massage therapists have chosen to open up their own businesses rather than work for someone else. What's sad is that the majority of therapists who attempt to sell their massage businesses fail to do so. In part, they don't know where to begin the process. Or they don't have the professional "tools" to carry out the process. Furthermore, they often discover their business has no equity in it, because they didn't develop that aspect of the business.

Selling your business can be an emotional experience. After all, you have spent much time and effort building up your business. It's probably one of your biggest accomplishments. The sale of your business can happen quickly if you have an interested buyer, or it can take a long time to find a buyer. Therefore, it is essential that you allow enough time for this process. Taking the necessary steps, as listed within this chapter, can help reduce the length of time.

There are some important considerations for you to address when thinking about selling your business. Like should you use a broker or sell it yourself? What is your business' worth? How do you prepare the business for sale? How will you find a buyer? And how should you advertise the business for sale? Let's examine each of these questions more closely.

BROKER VERSUS SELF

There are basically two ways to sell your business. You can (1) hire a business broker who will list your business for sale, market it, and then sell it, or (2) do all of the work yourself.

A business broker, like a real estate agent, will guide you in preparing the business for sale, market it for you, screen prospective buyers to see if they are serious buyers and financially qualified, and assist you at the closing. They are experts in the field who do all of the work for you, enabling you to focus your time and energy on your business. Their fee is earned only if the business sells, and is usually commissioned at around 10 percent of the sale price (not the listed price).

Selling your business by yourself will save you the cost of paying a fee to a business broker, which can amount to thousands of dollars, but you will have to do all of the work yourself. Unless you have done a lot of homework on how to sell a business, it will be the more difficult way to go. You will need to learn how to create a business offering page and a business prospectus, how to market the business for sale, and how to negotiate the sale when an offer is made. Once you have a buyer, you will need to know the definition of due diligence, escrow, and so forth. You will also need to hire an attorney to prepare important legal documents, which a broker would have provided.

Although I will discuss the basic outline to selling a business within this chapter, if you are determined to sell your business yourself, I recommend you read the book, *Selling Your Business Successfully*, by Rexford E. Umbenhaur III. This book will give you a more complete understanding with detailed scenarios on how you can sell your business without a business broker.

OFFERING PRICE

The offering price is the price for which you "offer" to accept in return for selling the business. But how do you arrive at the offering price? You could just tag a price on the business based on what you think it is worth, but a prospective buyer will want justification for your price. You will have to provide financial information that shows your business is worth your offering price.

One way to determine the value of your business is to hire a business broker to do a business valuation. This is strictly an opinion based on a detailed analysis of your business' worth, taking into consideration your prior income tax records, the business assets (such as furniture), the various means of business income (such as retail sales, independent contractors, and so forth), the amount of competition in your area, as well as other factors. Usually two or three different accounting formulas are used, then the average is taken to arrive at the business' value.

If you cannot find a business broker to do a valuation on your business, you can hire an accountant or use your own business accountant. They are also qualified to do a business valuation; however, they can be more conservative and may value your business lower than a business broker will.

Once you have a completed business valuation, you can use it as a guideline for establishing your offering price. Your offering price is often not the same as the sale price, which is the price you actually sell the business for. It is usually higher than the sale price, leaving room for negotiating. The sale price can sometimes be higher than the offering price, but that is rare. It can happen if two or more buyers are interested in purchasing the business at the same time.

In addition to deciding on an offering price, you will need to decide on the minimum amount of money you are willing to sell your business for. If, for example, your offering price is $100,000, you may decide to sell the business for a minimum of $80,000. Of course, you will not let any prospective buyers know your minimum acceptable offer. It's just good to have an idea in mind prior to negotiating the sale.

You will also have to decide how much of a down payment you would like and whether you will offer to finance any amount of the sale. Financing a portion of the sale will make it easier for buyers to purchase your business because they will need less money up front. In addition, it assures the buyer that you have faith in the success of your business, after you are gone. This information will be placed on your purchasing agreement, discussed later.

PRESENTATION OF YOUR BUSINESS

As it is with the sale of a home, your business must be ready to be presented to prospective buyers. This means all necessary repairs should be completed and the premises should be clean, organized, and ready to be viewed.

In addition, you will need to prepare both a business offering page and a business prospectus. If you are planning to hire a business broker to sell your business, you can count on the broker to prepare both of these documents; however, preparation of the business prospectus will cost a fee. If you plan to sell the business without a broker, you will need to learn how to create these documents yourself.

Business Offering Page

The business offering page is used to state the terms of the sale. (A sample is shown in the Appendix B, page 78.) It lists your offering price, the amount of down payment you are requesting, any seller financing offered, as well as a listing of the items included in the sale. This document is placed on the second page of the business prospectus, following the table of contents.

Business Prospectus

The business prospectus is a detailed analysis of your business. It offers core information regarding your business, including financial data to justify your offering price. It is typewritten and secured in a binder for presentation. The first page is the table of contents, followed by the business offering page, then the following four sections:

Section one begins with a summary of your business: (1) the business name, (2) location, (3) facilities and lease (Note: Your lease must be transferable.), (3) date of establishment, (4) business hours, (5) business highlights/key points, (6) reason for selling, (7) history of business, (8) business description and services, (9) staff, (10) marketing methods, (11) competition, (12) market/demand, and (13) future business expectations.

Section two is a typewritten listing of all the business assets and the value you have placed on each item.

Section three is your financial information. I recommend using copies of three to five years of income tax returns. You may need to add a footnote explaining any adjustments such as depreciation on equipment or a vehicle. Also include a one-year cash flow sheet that points out any expenses you take deductions on that are not absolutely necessary to run the business such as meals, contributions, personal health insurance, personal vehicle costs, and extra telephones such as cellular phones.

Section four includes any marketing materials you use such as a business logo, brochures, rate cards, a copy of your telephone directory advertisement, postcards you mail to clients, and so forth. You can also include any articles written about your business. You may want to include some photos of your business.

On the final page of the presentation package, list your contact information: name, address, telephone number, email address, and fax number.

MARKETING THE SALE

A large part of selling your business involves finding your target market. After all, to sell your business, you must reach the people who are willing to purchase it. But first you will need to prepare the information you will send to them. You will also need to write some short catchy blurbs (the highlights) about your business to place in classified advertising columns.

Business Acquisition Sheet

An important marketing tool used for advertising your business for sale is a business acquisition sheet. (A sample is shown in Appendix B, page 82.) Your broker, provided you have one, will prepare this for you. This is the advertising document for mailings and to give to anyone who inquires about purchasing your business. Within it you will find a description of the services the business offers, the history of the business, the reason the business is for sale, a description of the location and facility, the highlights of the business, and contact information for inquiries.

What it does not disclose is any personal financial information. That information will be divulged after the prospective buyer shows a sincere interest and signs a confidentiality warranty. It also does not mention the specific name of the business and address. The title of the business acquisition sheet should read "Massage Therapy Business for Sale." This will help keep the sale confidential. The last thing you want is for your clients to hear you are selling the business and to start looking for another therapist.

Confidentiality Warranty

Another form you will need prepared for marketing your business is called a confidentiality warranty. This warranty basically protects the confidentiality of the seller's personal financial business information. It also keeps the sale of the business quiet. The buyer promises to not disclose to anyone any of the financial information pertaining to the seller's business, without prior written permission. Written permission is sometimes acquired so the prospective buyer can show the financial information to an accountant for an opinion.

This legal document should be prepared for you by an attorney if you do not have a broker.

PROSPECTIVE BUYERS

Finding a buyer for your business can be a challenge. If you find your target market, however, it will save you time and money.

When I was in the process of selling my business, I had investors—and a variety of people who didn't know the first thing about running a massage therapy business—calling me. I quickly realized that the best candidate for purchasing my business would be a fellow massage therapist. After all, a large amount of my business' income was generated from my hands-on work. If someone bought my business and didn't take over my clientele, they would still earn income from the independent contractors and the sale of retail products and gift certificates, but their income potential would be sub-stantially less. Taking into consideration my offering price, it would hardly be worth it for a person who was not a massage therapist to purchase my business.

I also realized the best candidate for purchasing my business would need to hold a massage therapy license in my state in order to take over my clientele. Although a massage therapist who held a state license from another state or who had the proper qualifica-tions could apply for a license in my state, it would just take longer. This information helped me focus on my target market.

Once you've narrowed down your target market, you can start looking for a buyer. I would suggest beginning your marketing cam-paign within your own business. If you have independent contractors or employees working within your business, ask each of them sepa-rately if they are interested in purchasing your business. Since they already know the business well, they may be interested.

Otherwise, you will need to find the appropriate places to ad-vertise your business for sale. Depending on whether or not there are licensing requirements in your state, it would be best to first focus your advertising in areas within and surrounding your busi-ness, then branch out within your state. A local massage therapist who hasn't established a clientele yet would benefit from purchas-ing a well-established business. In addition, a massage therapist already licensed in your state who wishes to relocate within the state would also benefit from purchasing a thriving business. After focusing on marketing within your state, you can branch out to ad-joining states and so on.

To contact local massage therapists, you can mail them your business acquisition sheet. I also recommend sending this sheet to all of the massage therapy schools within your state and adjoining your state, asking them to post the advertisement. Some schools have their own newsletter and will want you to pay a small fee to advertise in it. After mailing your business acquisition sheet to each school, call them and see if they received the information and posted it, and if they have a newspaper you could advertise in.

Another marketing suggestion is to contact local spa or hair salons that may be interested in purchasing your business to add to their business.

If you are a member of any massage- or health-related associations, contact them to see where you can place advertisements. Many associations now have websites that host classified ads. Some also have professional journals or magazines where advertising in the classified section will reach thousands of massage therapists. You may also contact your association's state chapter and see if you can purchase a state mailing list to use for sending your business acquisition sheet to massage therapists.

If you have a broker, he or she will do all of the marketing for you at their expense. You will, however, benefit from gathering all of the marketing ideas and mailing lists for the broker. After all, you know your target market and how to reach them better than your broker does.

NEGOTIATING THE SALE

Once you have found an interested buyer, you will need to come to an agreement on the sale price. Your next move is to give the buyer a blank purchasing agreement, (A sample is in Appendix B, page 83.) which your attorney or broker prepares for you, and wait to receive a written offer. Within the document, there will be a stated period of time the purchaser has to accept your offer or make a counteroffer before the offer becomes null and void.

Another suggestion would be to add two purchasing agreements to the end of your Business Prospectus. The first agreement will be filled in with your offering price and terms of the sale. The second will be left blank for the buyer to make you a counteroffer.

You may receive the initial purchasing agreement back, signed with a deposit, or you may receive a counteroffer along with a deposit. If you receive a counteroffer, you can then choose to accept the offer or send another counteroffer back to the buyer along with their deposit. This is part of the negotiating experience, and hopefully you will come to an agreeable sale price.

Due Diligence and Escrow

After a sale price is agreed upon by both the buyer and the seller and the purchasing agreement is signed by both parties, due diligence and escrow begin. This is a period of time (usually 30 days) in which the buyer has the right to investigate your business records and observe your daily operations. The reason for due diligence is so that the buyer can verify the seller has not withheld important information and to verify the business records have not been misrepresented. If the buyer discovers any misrepresented information, the buyer can be released from obligation from the signed purchasing agreement and the pending sale can fall through.

During the due diligence period, the seller has the right to verify that the buyer has the finances to purchase the business. If you have a broker, he or she will do this step for you, although he or she may have already prequalified the buyer. To verify the buyer's finances, you can request the buyer's financial statement, a credit report, and/ or an approval note from the bank providing the loan.

Escrow means that the deposit on the purchasing agreement is held in trust by a third party. This is usually either your broker or attorney. The third party is responsible for handing over the deposit at the closing. Holding the deposit in escrow assures that neither the buyer nor the seller has control over the money during the due diligence period.

Closing

If you have reached this phase of selling your business, congratulations! The closing phase can be an exciting and emotional experience. You are about to sell the business you have worked so hard to build, and you are going to receive money for it! It's bittersweet.

In order for the closing to proceed smoothly, you must have an attorney assist you. Sometimes the attorney is shared by both the buyer and the seller, but I recommend you have your own attorney. Usually, the closing attorney(s) fees are split equally between the buyer and the seller and are outlined in the purchasing agreement.

Prior to the closing date, contact your attorney to see what you are required to bring to the closing. Sometimes, for example, you will bring a product inventory list, compiled that day. You may also need to bring a list of the business' assets. The attorney will use this list to calculate how much state sales tax the buyer will have to pay on the purchase of the business assets. A specific sales tax form needs to be filled out, which your attorney should provide. You should also request that your attorney send you a copy of all of the documents you will sign at the closing so you can review them.

Be prepared to sign a lot of legal documents at the closing. Some of the documents will include a bill of sale, a covenant not to compete form, a subordination of security agreement and note (if a loan is used for purchasing the business), a security agreement (if you are providing financing), and an assignment and assumption of lease form (if you are transferring your lease). If you have any questions, make certain you get them answered before signing any documents.

Plan on receiving a substantial check at the closing, including the deposit held in escrow. The attorney will deduct from the check your portion of the attorney fees and the broker's fee (if you have one). The attorney will create a statement of sale, showing the allocation of the sale price. Once all the documents are signed and the money is allocated, the closing is complete.

Be sure to plan a special celebration for your new greatest accomplishment!

Steps to Selling Your Business Successfully

- Be prepared
- Determine offering price
- Find your target market
- Market with business acquisition sheet
- Get signed confidentiality warranty
- Send business prospectus
- Negotiate sale price
- Obtain signed sale contract with deposit
- Due diligence and escrow
- Closing

Contacts and Considerations

RESOURCES

- American Massage Council, (800) 500-3930
- American Massage Therapy Association, (847) 864-0123
- Associated Bodywork and Massage Professionals, (800) 458-2267
- Get Physical Software, 15 East Putnam Avenue, Suite 376, Greenwich, CT 06830, (800) 622-0025, www.dancesoft.net
- Hemingway Publications, Inc., (815) 877-5590, www.heming waymassageproducts.com
- Holistic.com
- Information for People, (800) 754-9790, www.info4people.com
- International Massage Association, (540) 351-0800
- Island Software Co., 717 Lingco Drive, Richardson, TX 75081, (877) 384-0295, www.island softwareco.com
- Land Software, 5138 Fulton Street NW, Washington DC 20016, (202) 237-2733, www.landsw.com
- massage4life.com
- massagenet.com
- massagenetwork.com
- massageregister.com
- massageresource.com
- massageware.com, 5028 First Coast Highway, Fernandina Beach, FL 32034, (800) 520-8514, www.massageware.com
- My Receptionist, 409 Main Street, Eau Claire, WI 54701, (800) 686-0162, www.myreceptionist.com
- Onebody.com
- Staying In Touch: (877) 634-1010
- Time Trade Systems, Inc., 235 Bear Hill Road, Waltham, MA 02451, (781) 890-4808, www.timetrade.com

EMPLOYEES VERSUS INDEPENDENT CONTRACTORS

Employee	*Independent Contractor*
Follows set instructions on where, when, and how to perform work	Follows own individual instructions and performs work based on own procedures
Receives and/or is required to receive training	Skilled professional requiring no training to perform services
Provides essential services which meld into overall business operation	Work performed is not an "integral part," it is a "unique" service
Required to work set hours	Maintains control over own hours worked
Required to work on-site	Rents/leases location where work is performed and can simultaneously work elsewhere
Does not collect payment for services; instead receives paycheck from business owner	Receives direct payment for services
Tools and materials for services are provided by business	Supplies own tools and materials
May be required to wear appropriate attire	Has control over attire and a dress code or uniform cannot be mandated
May terminate relationship at any time	May terminate relationship only upon completion of contract or breach by other party

Sample Forms

SAMPLE BUSINESS CONTRACT

THIS AGREEMENT made by and between PROFESSIONAL MASSAGE ASSOCIATES, 7 Wells Street, Saratoga Springs, New York, hereinafter known as PMA and (independent contractor's full name), hereinafter known as Independent Contractor.

The parties above hereby agree as follows:

TERMS: The Independent Contractor has the use of one treatment room at PMA for the purpose of Professional Therapeutic Treatments at a rental fee of Thirteen ($13.00) Dollars per hour treatment, Nine ($9.00) Dollars per ½ hour treatment, and Nineteen ($19.00) Dollars per 1 ½ hour treatment. This room shall be made available to the Independent Contractor on specific hours as agreed between the parties.

PMA shall be responsible for supplying a massage table, sink, music system and music, soap, and paper towels, in each treatment room. The Independent Contractor shall supply, at its sole expense, all oils/lotions, blankets, and additional supplies and equipment necessary to provide the professional services.

The Independent Contractor shall work as an independent contractor, and is not and will not be an employee of PMA. Nothing contained in this Agreement shall be interpreted or construed to constitute the Independent Contractor as a partner, employee, or agent of PMA, nor shall either party have any authority to bind the other in any respect, it being intended that each shall remain an independent contractor responsible for his/her/its own actions.

INSURANCE: The Independent Contractor shall secure and have in effect liability insurance in an amount not less than $1,000,000.00, which provides for personal injury and wrongful death. The Independent Contractor shall be solely responsible for obtaining, maintaining, and paying all premiums for coverage for the entire duration of this Agreement, and will provide PMA with a current certificate of coverage.

The Independent Contractor agrees to indemnify and hold harmless PMA and Colleen Steigerwald, the owner, for any and all negligent or intentional acts or omissions of the Independent Contractor which result in personal injury, wrongful death or property damage.

LINENS: The Independent Contractor shall pay Fifty Five Cents ($.55) per sheet used, Fifty Cents ($.50) per large towel used, Twenty Cents ($.20) per small towel used, Thirty Cents ($.30) per pillow case used, Ten Cents ($.10) per washcloth used, and Forty Cents ($.40) per apron used, which will be added to the rent, due on the last day of each month.

PRODUCTS: PMA will purchase all retail products. The Independent Contractor will receive a 20% commission on all retail product she/he sells, which will be deducted from the monthly rental fee on the last day of each month.

FEES: All fees for services shall be paid directly to the Independent Contractor, with the exception of credit card transactions, which shall be paid to PMA, and 96% deducted by the Independent Contractor from the rent due on the last day of each month. A 4% credit card usage fee will be paid to PMA.

On the last calendar day of each month, the Independent Contractor will pay to PMA the total sum due to PMA for the usage of the room and linen service, in accordance with a log kept by the Independent Contractor. A late fee of Ten ($10.00) Dollars per day will be charged to the Independent Contractor for each day the rent is not paid.

DURATION: This is an ongoing Agreement, beginning _____, 20___.

(i) Either party may terminate this Agreement at any time by giving the other party written notice at least (30) days prior to the effective date of such termination.

(ii) If the Independent Contractor fails to give PMA thirty (30) days written notice of the termination of this Agreement, the Independent Contractor agrees to pay PMA the sum of Two Hundred Fifty ($250.00) Dollars immediately.

This Agreement contains the entire understanding of the parties and supersedes all previous verbal and written agreements. There are no other agreements, representations, or warranties not set forth herein.

The parties hereto have signed this Agreement on _____ day of _____, 20___.

PROFESSIONAL MASSAGE ASSOCIATES
BY: _____
COLLEEN STEIGERWALD, LMT

_____
INDEPENDENT CONTRACTOR

SAMPLE CLIENT INTAKE FORM

Name_____ Date _____

Street_____ City _____

State_____ Zip_____

Telephone (Home)_____ (Business) _____

Email address _____

Occupation_____ Date of birth _____

Referred by _____

Reason for therapeutic massage appointment _____
_____

When and how did this condition develop? _____
_____

Have you had surgery in the past few years? Explain? _____
_____

What vitamins, herbs and medications do you regularly take? _____
_____

Please check all of the following that currently apply to you:

____Allergies	____Tinnitus	____PMS
____Arthritis	____Ulcers	____Broken Bones
____Bursitis	____Fatigue	____Skin Disorders
____Cancer	____Severe Depression	____Stomach Disorders
____Diabetes	____Blood Clots	____Abdominal Hernia
____Edema	____Varicose Veins	____Herniated Disc
____Diarrhea	____Heart Conditions	____Neck Pain
____Constipation	____Low Blood Pressure	____Back Pain
____Sinusitis	____High Blood Pressure	____Chest Pain
____Headaches	____Shortness of Breath	____Sciatica
____Dizziness	____Poor Posture	____Scoliosis
____Numbness	____Respiratory Problems	____TMJ Syndrome
____Pregnant	____Contact Lenses	____Hearing Aid
____AIDS	____Menstrual Pain	____Exercise Regularly

Do you have any health conditions, not listed above? Explain _____
_____

How will payment for treatment be made?

   Cash_____ Check_____ Insurance_____

Who is responsible for the payment? _____

All information is strictly confidential and will only be released upon client's written request.

Client's signature _____

SAMPLE PRESS RELEASE

FOR IMMEDIATE RELEASE
Contact: Colleen Steigerwald, LMT, (518) 587-3827

Professional Massage Associates, located at 7 Wells Street, Saratoga
Springs, New York, is proud to announce Jennifer Greyson, LMT,
has joined the business. Jennifer, a graduate of the Fulton School of
Massage, is a New York State Licensed Massage Therapist. She has
advanced training in Cranio-Sacral Therapy and Neuromuscular
Therapy, and accepts insurance reimbursement for no-fault and
worker's compensation injuries. For more information or to schedule an appointment, call (518) 587-3827.

SAMPLE INTRODUCTION
LETTER TO PHYSICIANS

(Print on company letterhead)

Date

Dear Dr._____:

I am writing to introduce myself to you and to announce that I have recently opened a massage therapy business at 7 Wells Street in Saratoga Springs.

My name is Colleen Steigerwald. I am a New York State Licensed Massage Therapist who specializes in deep tissue massage, incorporating neuromuscular therapy and myofascial therapy techniques. I have advanced training in trigger point therapy, which is especially effective for treating neck and back injuries.

My business, Professional Massage Associates, includes a highly skilled, professional staff of five massage therapists, an acupuncturist, and an aesthetician. I have enclosed our brochure, with additional information, for your review. Please feel free to call me with any questions.

I look forward to meeting you and learning more about your business.

Yours in health,

Colleen. S. Steigerwald, LMT
Enclosure

SAMPLE BUSINESS OFFERING PAGE

Professional Massage Associates
7 Wells Street, Suite 101
Saratoga Springs, New York 12866

OFFERED FOR: $115,000
INVENTORY INCLUDED: $1,000
EARNEST DEPOSIT: $10,000
SELLER FINANCING: $30,000

TERMS: As a self-amortizing note to seller to be at 7.5% for 36 months. A monthly payment of approximately $933.19. Buyer may prepay all or part of the note without penalty. The note is to be secured by the tangible assets of the business.

TRAINING/CONSULTING: Seller offers to train and consult with buyer for a period of 30 days.

LEASE: Completely transferable upon proof of financial ability of buyer; Lease expires March 1, 2003.

OTHER CONDITIONS: The seller will provide the following specific assistance to buyer: (1) introduction to suppliers, customers, the landlord, building neighbors, and such other persons as may be necessary; (2) assistance in determining and ordering inventory, and will also recommend levels of inventory to be ordered and carried throughout the period; (3) assistance with hiring and training staff; (4) access to or copies of all relevant records as may be helpful to the profitable operation of the business; (5) assistance in determining an annual budget and cash flow schedule; (6) assistance and personal instruction in all aspects of operating the business including scheduling, staffing, inventory, cleaning, ordering, personnel supervision, the operation of all equipment, banking, relations with the landlord, and such other items as may be needed from time to time.

ASSETS INCLUDED IN SALE: A complete, attached hereto, listing of all business assets, as well as business reputation and goodwill. A complete list of customers and suppliers, and a transferable lease to the premises. A signed non-compete agreement.

ACCOUNTS RECEIVABLE INCLUDED IN SALE: None.

REAL ESTATE INCLUDED IN SALE: None, but the conclusion of an acceptable lease to the premises is a condition of this offer.

LIABILITIES TRANSFERRED OR ASSUMED: None.

SAMPLE MENU OF SERVICES

SIDE ONE
PROFESSIONAL MASSAGE ASSOCIATES

We warmly extend an invitation to you to make an appointment for yourself or someone you care about. Come experience a therapeutic treatment in a tranquil setting, by the hands of our highly qualified staff.

PROFESSIONAL SERVICES AND RATES
Professional Massage (30 min)	$ 35.00
Professional Massage (60 min)	$ 55.00
Pre-Natal Massage (60 min)	$ 55.00
European Facial (75 min)	$ 75.00
Specialized Facials	$40.00 - $70.00
Facial Waxing	$7.00 - $30.00
Foot Reflexology (60 min)	$ 55.00
Stone Therapy (90 min)	$100.00
(60 min)	$ 75.00
Acupuncture Treatment (60 min)	$ 60.00
Chinese Herbal Consult. (30 min)	$ 50.00
Initial Acupuncture (90 min)	$ 75.00

Appointments are Necessary
Open Monday thru Saturday

GIFT CERTIFICATES AVAILABLE

(INSERT MAP HERE)

PROFESSIONAL MASSAGE ASSOCIATES
7 Wells Street, Suite 101
Saratoga Springs, New York 12866
587-3827

SIDE TWO
Rejuvenate both body and spirit by choosing from an array of Eastern and Western methods of bodywork...

SWEDISH MASSAGE - A technique that incorporates long, gliding strokes, muscle-kneading and manipulation of "trigger points" to soothe sore muscles, stimulate the nervous system, and promote good health and relaxation.

*MEDICAL MASSAGE - Will aid in facilitating the healing process of a variety of medical conditions, such as bursitis, fibrositis, back & neck pain, whiplash, tendonitis, & TMJ. Some insurance coverage w/medical prescription.

PRE-NATAL MASSAGE - As your body changes, during pregnancy, this soothing massage relieves backaches, leg cramping, & sciatic pain. Reclaim your body for an hour, using our comfortable Prego pillow.

EUROPEAN FACIAL - An indepth skin analysis followed by cleansing, exfoliation, steam, extractions, facial massage and then mask. Hands and feet are massaged and placed in heated mitts. Eye cream is the final step.

SPECIALIZED FACIALS - Customized treatments to clear skin of underlying congestion due to build up, rehydrate dry and/or mature complexions, diminish fine lines, improve skin clarity, and assist the skin in its natural renewal process. ask our skin care expert for her recommendation.

FOOT REFLEXOLOGY - A ten minute herbal foot soak followed by a soothing therapeutic system of applying specific pressure points and massage techniques on the feet.

STONE THERAPY - Unique combinations of energy balancing techniques with massage using heated basalt stones. Tranquil, relaxing and therapeutic.

*ACUPUNCTURE AND CHINESE HERBAL MEDICINE - Capable of treating stress, pain & countless other ailments. It balances the body's energy system and stimulates the immune system. Some insurance coverage.
*No-Fault and Worker's Compensation Injuries Accepted
587-3827
PROFESSIONAL MASSAGE ASSOCIATES

SAMPLE REFERRAL PAD

PROFESSIONAL MASSAGE ASSOCIATES
7 Wells Street, Suite 101
Saratoga Springs, New York 12866
518-587-3827

Patient Name _____

Diagnosis/Impression _____

ICD-9 Diagnosis Code _____

I am referring the above mentioned patient to you for soft tissue manipulation/neuromuscular re-education therapy.

Prescribed Length of Treatment:

_____ times a week for _____ weeks

_____ times a month for _____ months

_____ treatments

_____   _____
Doctor's Signature   Date

_____
Doctor's Address and Phone #

In making this referral, the Doctor certifies that
Prescribed treatment is a medical necessity.

SAMPLE TELEPHONE DIRECTORY AD

PROFESSIONAL MASSAGE ASSOCIATES

Colleen Steigerwald LMT & Associates

- Immediate Pain Relief
- NYS Licensed Therapists
- Massages - Facials - Foot Reflexology
- Hot Stone Massage
- Acupuncturist/Chinese Medicine
- Accident Insurance & Others
- Gift Certificates / Visa & MC

587-3827
7 Wells Street, Saratoga

BUSINESS ACQUISITION SHEET

AVAILABLE FOR ACQUISITION
Profitable Massage Therapy Business with repeat clients
Northeastern New York

BUSINESS ACTIVITY:

THIS BUSINESS, FOUNDED IN 1993 BY ITS CURRENT OWNER, PROVIDES SEVERAL DISTINCT TYPES OF MASSAGE THERAPY: SWEDISH MASSAGE, MEDICAL MASSAGE, PRENATAL MASSAGE, FOOT REFLEXOLOGY; STONE THERAPY, FACIALS, ACUPUNCTURE AND CHINESE HERBAL MEDICINE TO A GROWING BASE OF SATISFIED CLIENTS. IT ALSO RETAILS PUREPRO AND PRESCRIPTIONS PLUS LINE OF PRODUCTS.

WHY BUY THIS BUSINESS?

THIS IS A WELL-ESTABLISHED, PROFITABLE, TURN-KEY OPPORTUNITY WITH A SOLID REPUTATION. IT IS COMPLETELY EQUIPPED, A GOING CONCERN, NICELY PROFITABLE AND THE BUYER(S) WILL BE RECEIVING INCOME FROM THE FIRST DAY.

HISTORY:

THE 8-YEAR OLD BUSINESS HAS GROWN IN BOTH CUSTOMER BASE AND IN REPUTATION. THE SATISFIED CLIENT BASE CONTAINS A SUBSTANTIAL NUMBER OF RETURN CUSTOMERS. THE THERAPISTS ARE ALL INDEPENDENT CONTRACTORS SO THERE ARE NO EMPLOYEE ISSUES. THE BUSINESS' REPUTATION HAS GROWN TO THE POINT THAT IT RECEIVES REFERRALS FROM DOCTORS AND OTHER MEDICAL PROFESSIONALS FOR VARIOUS TYPES OF MASSAGE THERAPY, INCLUDING THAT FOR WORKMAN'S COMPENSATION AND OTHER INSURANCE MATTERS.

REASON FOR SALE:

THE OWNER HAS DECIDED TO MARRY AND TO RELOCATE OUT-OF-STATE.

FACILITIES:

THE BUSINESS HAS A TRANSFERRABLE LEASE, RENEWABLE ALSO, IN A PROFESSIONAL BUILDING NEAR DOWNTOWN AND THE CITY CENTER. THE BUSINESS ITSELF HAS A WARM, INVITING LOOK AND IS FULLY EQUIPPED. THE BUILDING HAS SUPERB PARKING AND FULL HANDICAP ACCESS.

Acquisition Highlights

- *SOLIDLY PROFITABLE.*
- *SUPERB REPUTATION.*
- *COMPLETELY TURNKEY.*
- *COMPLETE RETAIL FILES AND SYSTEMS.*
- *SIGNIFICANT REPEAT BUSINESS WITH REGULAR CUSTOMERS FROM SEVERAL STATES.*
- *REASONABLE PRICE: TERMS INCLUDE POSSIBILITY OF OWNER FINANCING.*
- *COMPLETE CUSTOMER AND BUSINESS FILES.*
- *OWNER WILL INTRODUCE BUYER(S) TO CUSTOMERS AND ALL SUPPLIERS.*
- *OWNER WILL TRAIN BUYER(S).*
- *STAFF OF THERAPISTS HAS INDICATED DESIRE TO REMAIN WITH NEW OWNER.*

For further Information, contact the Broker:

PURCHASING AGREEMENT

OFFER TO PURCHASE AND SALE OF ASSETS

This Offer to Purchase made as of the date of execution hereof by and between _____, hereinafter referred to as Buyer, and _____, hereinafter referred to as Seller, and **Garrett, Jones and Flushing, Inc.**, hereinafter referred to as Broker.

In consideration of the mutual covenants and promises herein contained, and for other good and valuable consideration, the receipt and sufficiency of which is hereby acknowledged, the parties hereto agree as follows:

1.01 Buyer hereby offers to purchase substantially all of the tangible and intangible assets and business known as _____ and described as follows:

    (a) Location _____
    (b) Ownership _____
    (c) Form of Ownership: D.B.A.____ S Corp____ C Corp____
                        Partnership____ Other____

1.02 As consideration for the purchase of said business, as above described, Buyer shall pay to Seller the following amounts on the terms and conditions:

    (a) Full Sales Price _____

    (b) Down Payment _____
                          (Cash or Certified Funds only)

    (c) Seller financing _____

    (d) Terms _____

    (e) Other Conditions _____

    (f) Assets included in the sale _____

    (g) Accounts Receivable included in sale _____

    (h) Real estate included in sale _____

    (i) Liabilities transferred or assumed _____

1.03 The full purchase price shall include inventory of $_____ at Sellers cost. If the actual amount at closing is different, the variance shall be adjusted by the parties outside escrow or by adjusting the down payment or note to Seller.

1.04 Upon the execution hereof, Buyer has paid to Broker, or other party, as escrow agent, the amount of $_____. This money shall constitute an earnest money deposit toward the transaction contemplated hereby, and shall apply as a credit against the down payment at the closing hereof, subject to the provisions of Section 4.01 and 4.02 below. Any non-certified fund deposit shall be replaced with certified funds upon satisfactory completion of Section 3.02 below.

1.05 All earnest money deposits shall be held by Broker who, at its option, may hold Buyer's deposit in an uncashed form until this agreement has been signed by Seller or it may be deposited in a segregated escrow account upon receipt.

1.06 Broker shall have no liability to any party for any actions it takes as escrow agent hereunder, unless it shall be found to have acted with gross negligence or willful misconduct. Notwithstanding the foregoing, Broker shall have no liability under such circumstances for any action or omission that is taken or made in good faith, and believed by Broker to be authorized or within the rights and power conferred upon Broker by this agreement.

1.07 The following adjustments and prorations shall be made at closing (if none, write 'none'):

1.08 Seller and/or Landlord shall deliver to Buyer an acceptable lease or lease assignment as per current terms and conditions, if applicable. This is to be handled outside of escrow.

1.09 Seller warrants that at the time of closing, all equipment will be in working order and that the premises will pass all inspections necessary to conduct such business.

1.10 Seller warrants that it has a good, clear and recorded, marketable title to the business being sold except as may be noted herein.

2.01 The execution hereof by Seller shall constitute the Seller's acceptance of the purchase price and the terms and conditions of sale set forth herein above. Upon the closing (as defined in Section 5.02 below) of the transaction contemplated hereby, Seller shall execute and deliver to the Buyer such bills of sale with full warranties, assignments of instruments and such other documentation as shall be necessary to vest in the Buyer good and marketable title to the business free and clear of any and all liens and encumbrances, except those expressly provided above.

3.01 If required, the Buyer shall be responsible for giving notice of the transfer to the creditors listed in the Seller's list of creditors, and take such other action as may be necessary to protect Buyer pursuant to the Bulk Transfer provisions of the Uniform Commercial Code of _____ State.

3.02 This Offer to Purchase is subject to a satisfactory due diligence review of the Books, Records, and Operations of the business by the Buyer and/or his agents. Seller shall provide access to same during normal business hours. Buyer shall have _____ days to complete this review. During this due diligence review, Buyer will not contact any customers or suppliers without Seller's prior approval and arrangements, for visit or other contact.

3.03 Seller shall enter into a Covenant Not to Compete in this type of business for a period of _____ ( ) years within the bounds of the following area:

If Seller is a Corporation, all shareholders of the Corporation shall sign and agree to the Covenant Not To Compete.

4.01 In the event that this Offer to Purchase is accepted by the Seller, but the sale contemplated hereby is not concluded on the closing date as stated below, unless an extension is agreed upon in writing by all parties, due to the failure of Seller to meet the terms and conditions of this Offer to Purchase and in the absence of any fault on the part of the Buyer, then Broker shall return to Purchaser the entire earnest money deposit.

4.02 Buyer agrees that if he should fail or refuse to complete this transaction after acceptance by the Seller and all contingencies have been satisfied, then any funds or deposit will be at the Broker's option forfeited and shall be split equally between the Broker and the Seller by the Escrow Agent.

5.01 The closing date shall be on or before _____, at the offices of_____, located at _____. Closing cost shall be shared equally by Seller and Buyer. Additionally, fees paid by the Buyer to his Attorney for actual attendance at the closing shall be shared equally by each party.

5.02 The closing of the transaction contemplated hereby shall be defined as the execution by Seller and Buyer of those documents that shall transfer title of the business and asset's subject hereof from the Seller to the Buyer.

6.01 Time is of the essence of this Offer to Purchase.

6.02 Broker shall bear no liability to either Buyer or Seller in the event of the failure of either Buyer or Seller to fulfill the obligations imposed hereby.

7.01 If the Seller fails to accept this agreement by 6:00 p.m._____, 200__, then the Buyer may revoke this agreement and deposit may be returned by Broker to Buyer.

7.02 To the extent that this Offer to Purchase concerns some of the same subject matter as a Previous Listing Commission Agreement, this Offer to Purchase shall be an addendum to such Agreement between the Seller and Broker, and the terms and provisions of the two instruments shall be reconciled and construed accordingly, and this Offer to Purchase shall not constitute nor be construed to be an expressed or implied limitation or termination of such Previous Agreement.

7.03 Any party to this Offer to Purchase shall be entitled to obtain specific performance of this Agreement as a remedy cumulative to any other remedy at law, in equity, by statute or by contract.

7.04 This document, and any other exhibits or addenda attached hereto and signed by the parties, contains the entire understanding of the parties and there are no oral agreements, understandings, or representations relied upon by the parties. Any modifications must be in writing and signed by all parties. Should there be any conflict between the provisions of this Offer to Purchase and Sale of Assets and any escrow instructions issued pursuant hereto, the provisions of this Offer to Purchase and Sale of Assets shall control.

7.05 Buyer agrees to hold in confidence and not to disclose or use for Buyer's own benefit any confidential or proprietary information received from Seller or its business during the 'Due Diligence' review for a period of three (3) years. Buyer's commitment shall not apply to:

(a) Information already known when received;
(b) Information in the public domain when received or thereinafter in the public domain through sources other than Buyer;
(c) Information lawfully obtained from a third party not subject to confidentiality obligation to Seller, or
(d) Information developed independently by personnel in Buyer's organization who did not have access to Seller's information.

Buyer agrees to restrict access to Seller's information to persons in Buyer's organization who have a need to know, and are subject to secrecy under the terms and conditions of the Buyer's Confidentiality and Warranty Agreement already undertaken by Buyer. If negotiations are discontinued or the sale does not close for any reason, Buyer will return all documents furnished to Buyer by Seller and/or Broker(s), and will keep no copies.

7.06 No public announcement of this Offer to Purchase shall be made without Seller's approval and Buyer's approval.

7.07 If the contemplated sale of the business does not close for any reason, Seller and Buyer shall bear their own expenses and have no further liability or obligation to each other.

7.08 Buyer and Seller fully agree and recognize that each was introduced to the other and that the contemplated execution of this Offer to Purchase and Sale of Assets was caused through the efforts of Broker. The parties also fully agree that Seller shall remain fully responsible for the payment of Broker's commission due and owing at closing as a result of this transaction, in accordance with the Broker's Listing Agreement.

7.09 Buyer understands and agrees that an allocation agreement of the sale price to the assets sold will have to be executed on IRS Form 8594 (Asset Acquisition Statement) when the sale closes, in order to establish Seller's tax and Buyer's basis for the transaction. Such allocation is based on fair market value. It is most strongly recommended by Broker that a CPA be consulted before executing this important document.

7.10 The Buyer shall be responsible for payment of all sales taxes at closing. If the _New York_ State Department of Taxation subsequently determines that additional sales taxes are payable, the Buyer shall pay same immediately.

7.11 Buyer understands that Seller and Broker have agreed that in the event any litigation is instituted to collect any sum due Broker or to enforce or to interpret any of the provisions of this Offer to purchase and Sale of Assets, the prevailing party or parties shall be entitled to recover from the other(s) their reasonable attorney's fees and court costs, including appeals, as determined by the court in such action or suit. Broker and Seller have further agreed that any and all disputes between these parties or their privities shall be resolved exclusively by the American Arbitration Association in the city nearest to Seller where such an Association exists and be covered by the Commercial Arbitration Rules of the American Arbitration Association. Seller and Broker agree to be bound by the results therein, which shall be entered into a court of competent jurisdiction. The expenses of arbitration conducted pursuant to this subparagraph shall be borne by the parties in such proportion as the arbitrator shall decide.

7.12 Broker hereby fully discloses and Buyer and Seller understand and acknowledge that Broker provides Business Valuation services in addition to Business Brokerage and other business services. In that capacity Broker may have provided a Business Valuation on the Business which is the subject of this particular Offer to Purchase and Sale of Assets. In that instance, Broker's compensation earned as a result of the sale of this particular Business may depend in a large part on the results of that Business Valuation. In conducting a Business Valuation, broker relies principally on the representations of the Seller without having independently audited or otherwise investigated the accuracy of those representations. Broker conducts Business Valuation activity in an independent and honest fashion, but is encouraged by the ethics of the profession to fully disclose to Buyer, Seller and other interested parties this possible conflict of interest.

7.13 Contingencies: (if none, write 'None') _____.
This provision does not survive the closing.

7.14 THIS IS A LEGALLY BINDING DOCUMENT. READ IT CAREFULLY. FOR YOUR PROTECTION AND IN PARTICULAR IF YOU DO NOT UNDERSTAND IT OR ANY PART OF IT, CONSULT AN ATTORNEY. Garrett, Jones and Flushing, Inc. cannot furnish personal counsel or advice or answer questions or inquiries that involve interpretations of law. Broker is required to submit all bona fide written offers to Seller.

Agreed to and Executed this _____ day of _____, 200__ . Receipt of a copy of this document is acknowledged by all signatories.

_____   _____
BUYER   SELLER

By: _____   By: _____
Title: _____   Title: _____
Address: _____   Address: _____

_____   _____
Telephone: _____   Telephone: _____

BROKER:
Garrett, Jones and Flushing, Inc.   By: James B Garrett

ABOUT THE AUTHOR

Colleen (Steigerwald) Holloway, LMT, is a workshop facilitator, business consultant, author, and successful business owner since 1993. Her profitable massage therapy business recently sold for six figures.

A 1991 graduate of the New Center for Holistic Health, Education and Research, Colleen also holds an associate degree in business.

Colleen is a member of the American Massage Therapy Association, formerly holding positions as New York State Education Chairperson, New York State Annual Convention Speaker Chairperson, and New York State Delegate.

Becoming an expert in the insurance field, she has taught insurance reimbursement seminars for over nine years, throughout New York State. Successfully winning a no-fault insurance arbitration ruling, Colleen set precedence for all New York State licensed massage therapists to receive no-fault insurance reimbursement.

Having hands-on experience as both a massage therapist and a business owner, Colleen hopes to help her colleagues to achieve their professional business goals, while following their passion for massage.